I0085285

Angel
of Compassion

Angel of Compassion

Mike Johnson

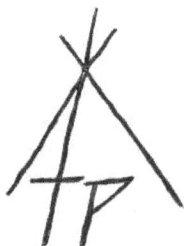

TP Press
An Imprint of Lasavia Publishing Ltd.
Auckland, New Zealand

www.lasavia.co.nz

Copyright © Mike Johnson, 2018.

All rights reserved. Artworks reproduced in this publication are the intellectual property of the artists that have created them. Other than artwork in the public domain no part of this publication may be reproduced, distributed, or transmitted in any form or by any means, including photocopying, recording, or other electronic or mechanical methods, without the prior written permission of the publisher, except in the case of brief quotations embodied in critical reviews and certain other noncommercial uses permitted by copyright law.

ISBN: 978-0-9941015-3-2

To my family, for their love and forbearance

Preface to the 2018 edition

A huge debt of gratitude is owed by the author to Mahina Marshall who put together the 2013 edition of this book. At the time, neither of us fully appreciated the challenge involved in putting together the text, the side texts and the images. A further debt of gratitude is owed to Daniela Gast for building on the foundation laid by Mahina to produce this 2018 edition. An additional thanks to all the artists who have generously allowed their work to be used in this publication.

Preface

The following is a transcription from a handwritten notebook called the 'Moleskin Notebook', begun on Monday October 4 soon after I came out of Auckland City Hospital, and finished on October 21, 2013. My thanks to Deborah Williams for taking dictation over a patchy Skype line, and inserting the images. The text has been corrected and lightly edited.

This is not so much a story as a report from experience. I have never written this way as I have never been able to find a voice for such a project, never perhaps needed one. All my voices have been fictional, all my codes of that journey, and the roads my characters travelled. Nor had I handwritten anything much since I was a child. My semi-dyslexic struggle with a familiar HB pencil and the creamy empty pages of my precious Moleskin Notebook, was a constant reminder of the first efforts I made to put thoughts into words on paper. In many ways it felt like the first thing I'd ever written.

I didn't choose to write this way for that reason or any other; I simply didn't have the physical strength to sit at the keyboard, but found I could prop myself up with pencil and notebook. I could keep writing. This time I wanted to relate what happened to me, not one of my characters, in my own voice. I still wonder if such a thing is possible.

Note: the boxed passages were originally conceived as sidebar stories. These were theoretical asides and bits of thought that did not belong in the main narrative. They arose because, in the Moleskin Notebook, I wrote on one side of the pages only, leaving blank facing pages which I began to fill with doodles, comments and illustrations.

Mike Johnson
December 8, 2013.

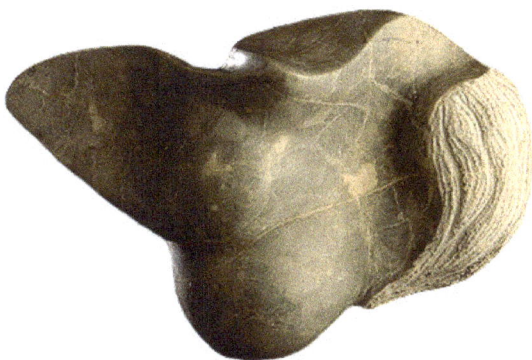

The Angel of Compassion

An Original Artwork by Sharon Gainsburg

Every Angel brings terror

Rainer Maria Rilke

1

Cards on the Table

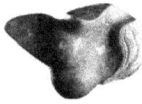

Let the cards fall where they may
Every dog will have its day

There is an angel of compassion hovering above Auckland hospital. That angel has its work cut out for it. I wonder, if among the angelic orders, they have rosters, shifts, twelve hours on and twelve hours off the way the nurses do in the building below. I hope so. Terrible to think of a lone angel of compassion serving a single shift for all eternity. That would grow wearying, even for an angel; it might come to seem more like a punishment than a vocation of joy.

I know there is such an angel, whatever the terms of its duty, because I have met it. Not in its pure form of existence, which would be impossible, as we would be consumed in that overwhelming existence, expire of terror in its arms as Rilke predicted, but rather in a very ordinary human form, the nature of which I did not immediately recognise.

I didn't go to Auckland hospital to meet any angel, rather to get a diagnosis for an abdominal pain, a flare-up I suspected of an ancient 'irritable bowel' I picked up in India in the '70s and never quite left behind. In that respect, the infamous Delhi Belly I believe still plagues visitors to that chaotic continent is a little bit like a memory – one that never lets go.

Moreover, I imagined that these abdominal pains were the result of standing a little too close to the freezer where we kept, or attempted to keep, our Mövenpick chocolate ice cream, surely the best if the most thoroughly overpriced chocolate ice-cream on the market. Dark chocolate, dairy and sugar! Ah!

Probably, I was so addicted to ice-cream because, two years before, I gave up the booze (or rather the booze gave me up) and I was craving sugar. Alcohol addiction, I have read, is merely an adult form of our great cultural addiction to sugar, one that we assiduously cultivate in our children. None of this was of any great interest to me at the time, and the abdominal pains not much more than a nuisance that wouldn't go away. My regular doctor, who I am calling Janet for the sake of this narrative, was away and I got to see a locum who became very concerned after prodding at my tender belly, and even more concerned at the news that one of my daughters, Sophia, had Crohn's disease at the tender age of 21 and that my mother had died of stomach cancer.

I have wondered since if things might not have turned out very differently if I had seen my regular doctor.

At the end of the consultation, the locum laid out the possibilities for me, which I imagined as cards on a card table, one of those fold-out card tables with a smooth, velvety green top. The first card was inflammatory bowel disease (IBD). This card could replicate into two cards, either Crohn's itself or diverticulitis, an inflammation or infection of the marble sized pockets that often develop on the bowel, a condition known as diverticulosis. There are other more obscure forms of IBD that might have to be put on the table later.

The second card was called bowel cancer, and of course we hoped it wasn't that. However, a certain dread began to affect me as soon as the card was placed on the table. If Crohn's was the Ace of Spades, cancer was the Joker.

I was sixty-six. 'Clickety-click,' I said jokingly to my brother on my birthday. The older you get, the more likely your number is to come up on the great roulette wheel of cancer. Cancer, in that respect, is not merely the quintessential illness of our time and our self-consuming culture, it is an apt metaphor for the crazy gamble we are taking with our life and all life around us. Our response when challenged on this is more likely to be to double down – double or nothing!

She ordered blood tests and a faeces test.

When I got home I looked into the mirror. I looked fit and healthy. I was lean, active, and working at my job as lecturer and creative writing teacher as well as working on my own writing. I could walk two or three kilometres without turning a hair. I didn't look clickety-click, I swear. When I looked in the mirror a comparatively youthful, bright-eyed man stared back at me. Bright-eyed and bushy tailed!

'All this is bullshit,' the image in the mirror said to me.

And so it seemed as I went for a walk on my beloved Waiheke Island. Thirty years I'd lived here, and the ground thudded reassuringly against my feet. I found myself on Palm Beach, carrying my shoes and feeling the wet sand squelch up between my toes. Palm Beach is a family sized beach, and we'd often come here when the kids were young. I didn't feel any different now to what I felt then, not inside.

Despite the niggling abdominal pain, already subsiding, I thought, I felt good. Walking felt good. And the island, in the pale wintery light had never looked better.

A couple of days later the results came back. Blood was discovered in one of the three faeces samples. My red blood cell count was way down. My haemoglobin levels were way down. I was becoming anaemic. Anaemia can be caused by loss of blood, and the loss of dark blood may not be recognised.

On the strength of the doctor's concern, backed up by my own doctor when she returned, I agreed to a colonoscopy, a highly unpleasant procedure in which a miniature camera is inserted through the anus and snaked up into the bowel as far as the opening to the small intestine. Readers who have had one of these clever procedures would probably agree that a colonoscopy is not something you rush gladly off to have. Those who had done this assured me that the procedure itself was uncomfortable rather than painful, that the worst part of it was drinking three litres of that awful gunk you must have in order to clear your bowels, so that the camera can actually see something other than shit.

Nothing anybody said had prepared me for the reality of what happened that day.

On the day of the great event, my wife Leila and I went to Auckland to spend the morning at Sophia's place on the North Shore, for the four hour drinking of the gunk ceremony, stuff quite as vile as everybody had said. By the time I was onto the third litre, I was beginning to have serious doubts. WTF!

I don't remember much about the taxi ride to the hospital (other than it cost me $40) or finding the right department, or putting on one of those humiliating gowns that opens at the back for easy access, but I do remember being briefed by a nurse who

HOW TO PUT ON A HOSPITAL GOWN

Place gown on as you would a coat

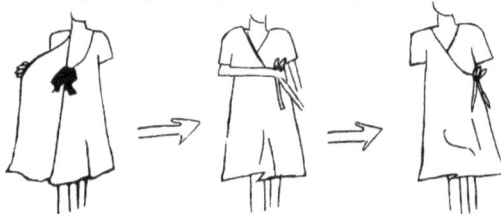

A quick snap of the infamous 'gown guide'

had a checklist of questions to ask – did I have any allergies, was I suffering this or that illness? A gentle Polynesian woman with a kind face.

I did my best to make light of the proceedings, and enjoyed jiving a little with the nurse, but my bonhomie quickly wore off after being wheeled into the procedure room. There was the gentle nurse, another nurse, and a man with his back to me sitting at a computer. The nurses proceeded to stick a little screw device into a vein on my left arm, an oxygen flow into my nose, and soon a soothing, presumably reassuring drug was flowing into my veins. I was not reassured. I thought I must look like a sick person, or the way a sick person looks on TV – tubes in, tubes out. Soon there would be another kind of tube in, and not one you'll see on TV.

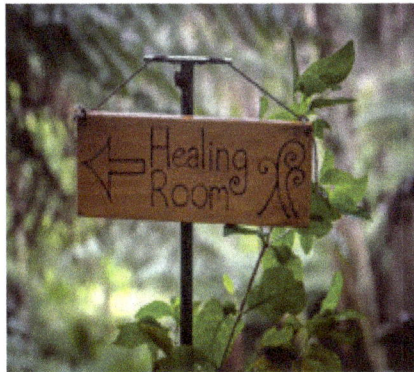

The man at the computer finally got up and came over to the bed. He introduced himself as the doctor who would perform the ritual of ass and camera. At that inappropriate moment I remembered my visit to Leila in her healing room on our Waiheke property, and what she had seen inside my bowel. To forestall a thousand questions to which there are no answers, I'll simply state that my wife is a seer, in the exciting and traditional sense of the word. A clairvoyant.

My original ready agreement to have a colonoscopy was not solely due to the concern of my own GP, Janet, that we get things cleared up as quickly as possible, but Leila's vision of a pulsing point somewhere in the bowel. She saw it on the right side and it did not look at all pleasant. This pulsing spot worried me as much as anything the doctors had said. I didn't like the sound of it. Leila saw 'healing forces' active around it and she herself was able to do 'a little work' on it. I thought of that pulsing spot as I looked up at the doctor, a man in his early forties maybe, brisk and confident, and wondered if the world of the seer and the

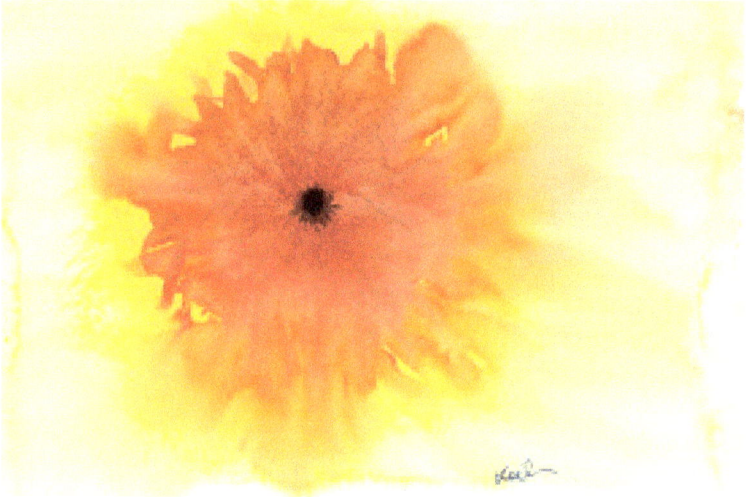

What Leila saw

world of the scientist, who was really just another kind of seer, would meet, and if this man might not see in his camera what Leila saw in her mind's eye. But did I really want him to? I had no investment in proving Leila right. I wanted her to be wrong. No

> *What does it mean when a writer assures you that a particular story is true or based on true events? Does it mean that other stories which offer no such assurance are false or based on false events?*
> *Humbug! Smoke and mirrors! A story is a story and a story is nothing more or less than that.*

one was more sceptical than me at that moment.

As events transpired, I would not get a satisfactory answer.

I became aware, once the camera had begun its invasion of my body on the end of a very thin tube, that all was not well. Houston had a problem.

Terse words were spoken between the doctor and the nurse. The oddity and discomfort I was warned about gave way to pain – sharp jabs of it. I began to twist and writhe on the bed. The gentle nurse with the kind face held me down.

When the pain got worse, the doctor ordered the nurse to feed more drugs into the drip. I was grateful to hear the news but it didn't make any difference. The pain got worse. For a second time the doctor upped the drug dose.

Briefly, the doctor explained that he was having problems getting the camera around the 'Sigmoid'. I thought he said Sigmund, which seemed pretty hilarious. This whole thing is inconveniently Freudian anyway, sticking things up people's bums. So he kept trying and still couldn't negotiate the Sigmund.

After a few minutes he stopped and announced that he would use the 'kiddy version', which was narrower and more flexible.

Good grief, they do this to kids! I thought, as I turned obediently on my side.

Further pain and probing ensued before the doctor finally abandoned the process. He'd moved from brief and business-like to terse to pissed off. Had I not been co-operating properly? I wondered. He explained, as I was being wheeled out, that I had a severe case of diverticulosis which had caused a 'hardening' in the bowel wall.

Because of this he'd had to abandon the colonoscopy.

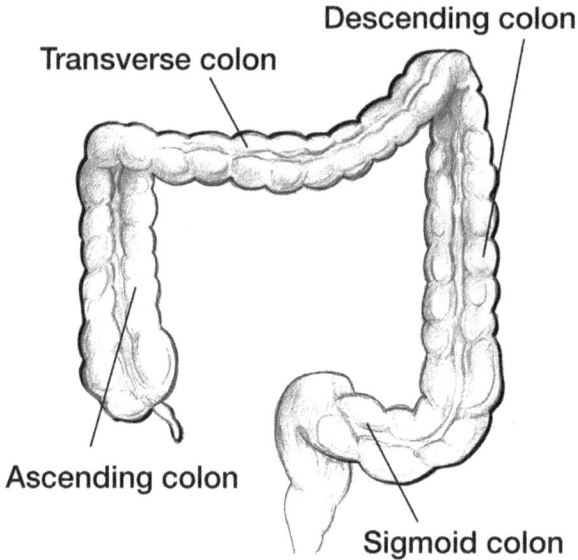

Descending colon

Transverse colon

Ascending colon

Sigmoid colon

Sigmoid Colon

On Probing

I have often wondered where the urban legend or cultural myth of alien abduction originated. The victim is removed from the planet and placed in a strange cold alien environment. Oddly hairless beings surround the victim, who is now helpless on a table or flat surface, and who is subjected to all kinds of indignities, anal probing in particular.

I say look no further than fear of invasive medical procedures for the source of these stories. Has anyone done a survey to find out how many abduction victims have had colonoscopies, or some like procedure?

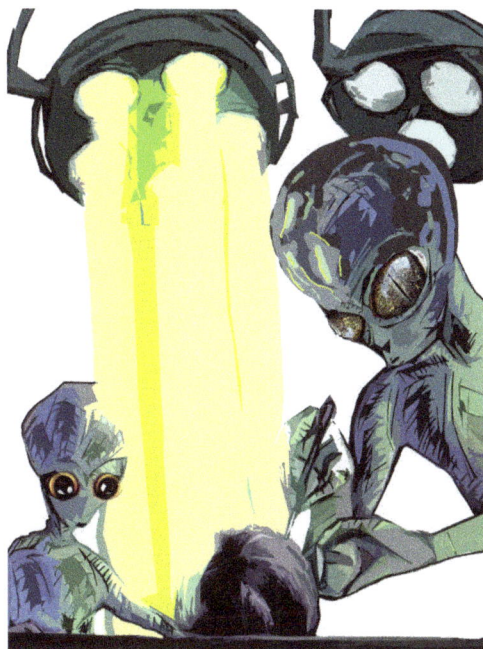

2

Across the Threshold

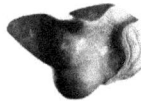

*For Beauty is nothing but the beginning of
terror we can barely endure*

Rainer Maria Rilke

This failed colonoscopy probably represented the high point in
my relations with the medical profession.

After all, the doctor might have been miffed at his failure to
complete the procedure but I had at least a diagnosis – one of
the cards that the locum had placed in front of me on that first
visit: diverticulosis a bowel condition which can at any moment
flare up into diverticulitis, an inflammation or infection of the
diverticula.

These were not words I could pronounce but at least I could
understand them.

One card face up.

According to the usual Google sources, some five to ten
percent of colonoscopies fail, mostly because of an obstruction
in the bowel, usually a cancerous tumour. I read all about it the
day afterwards. A blogosphere of various horror stories, mine
relatively minor. In some cases the procedure ruptured the wall

of the colon causing a serious crisis. Even death can result.

My GP Janet was not amused by this turn of events, which I had come to view with a certain perverse pride – as if my body had put up an underground act of resistance.

Janet had other things on her mind. Not only the worsening anaemia, but my blood pressure was now dropping to hell. For many years I had been fighting hypertension or high blood pressure and was on several blood pressure medications. Now we had some bizarrely low readings and I started having scary vertigo spells, possibly a side effect of low blood pressure. Janet started taking me off blood pressure meds. At the same time my weight was dropping, and I didn't have that much weight to lose; normally clocking in around seventy kilos I'd dropped to sixty-five and was still dropping. Worse, blood had shown up in one stool sample out of three. Called invisible blood, as it can't be seen.

While the original abdominal pain had subsided – mostly I believe due to Sophia's special Crohn's version of the Paleo diet –

The paleolithic diet (abbreviated paleo diet or paleodiet), also popularly referred to as the caveman diet, Stone Age diet and hunter-gatherer diet, is a modern nutritional plan based on the presumed ancient diet of wild plants and animals that various hominid species habitually consumed during the Paleolithic era — a period of about 2.5 million years which ended around 10,000 years ago with the development of agriculture and grain-based diets.

In common usage, the term "paleolithic diet" can also refer to actual ancestral human diets, insofar as these can be reconstructed. Centered on commonly available modern foods, the contemporary "Paleolithic diet" consists mainly of fish, grass-fed pasture raised meats, vegetables, fruit, fungi, roots, and nuts, and excludes grains, legumes, dairy products, potatoes, refined salt, refined sugar, and processed oils.

Janet was not convinced that things had returned to normal, and neither was I.

As Janet explained it, given the failure of the colonoscopy – which she described as a rare event, and one she'd never personally witnessed despite what I'd read on the net – the next best thing was a virtual colonoscopy. A CAT scan or CT scan is a sophisticated X-ray machine able to build up three dimensional images of whatever it sees. If the CT scan is so effective, why isn't it used before giving colonoscopies? I wondered. Seems less invasive.

Whatever, Janet began to spend time on the phone arguing that my case merited swift attention rather than being consigned to a long waiting list. She spoke rapidly to the movers and shakers at

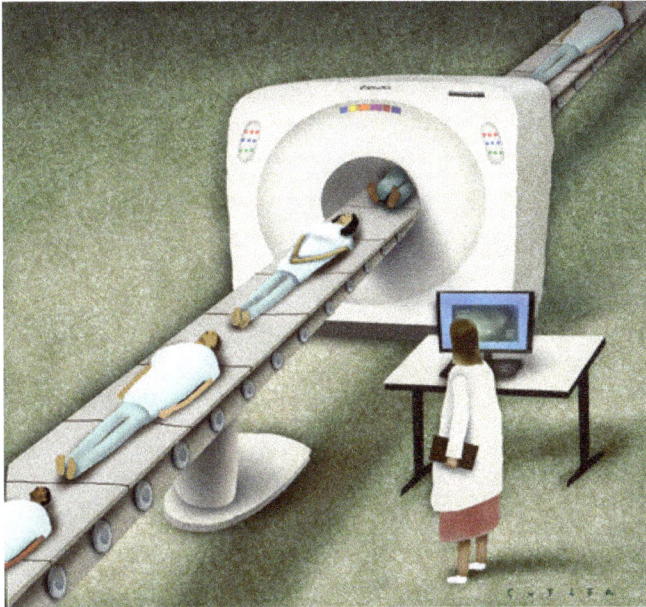

The CT Scanner in all its glory

Auckland Hospital, 'registrars' she called them, making her pitch, stressing my age, my family history, failed colonoscopy, blood show in stools, my ongoing anaemia, weight loss… to hear her talk you'd think I was a walking compendium of illness.

It was the failed colonoscopy that bugged the medical profession. Nobody knew what lay beyond the Sigmund. It was an uncharted, unconquered place. Any kind of abomination might lie there. A tumour, for example.

I had been thinking the same thing myself, and of the pulsing point Leila had seen. Cancer is a sneaky illness: it thrives in dark hidden places, biding its time before launching copies of itself into the bloodstream in search of further hidden places…

I made a return visit to the mirror to check out that lean, active, bright-eyed man who'd make jokes with his brother about being clickety-click. He was there but his eyes didn't look quite the same. It took me a while to understand fear. Fear can be sneaky too. But look at how I'd grasped for her Crohn's version of the Paleo diet as if it were the answer to everything. Crohn's was one of the cards the locum had originally put on the table. Only the

---

Sophia's Paleo Diet

No grains. OMG! Not just no gluten, but no grains of any kind, unless sprouted.

No nightshade family. OMG! I adored tomatoes and potatoes in equal measure.

No eggs. OMG! I was a two poached eggs a day on toast man.

No sugar. OK! OK! I get it.

No dairy products. Not even yoghurt. OK! I give up!

No legumes – unless sprouted. Farewell refried beans. Or any kind of beans.

The Menu: Meat, fish, kumara, coconut products, lashings of vegetables of all kinds, nuts and seeds (if thoroughly soaked), fresh fruit, especially bananas (but watch out for nature's candy!)

---

diverticulosis was face up, Crohn's and the Joker, cancer, were still face down. Having diverticulosis didn't exclude Crohn's, I could be looking at both cards face up on the table.

But it wasn't just that. I found in my daughter an inspiration. She had fought her Crohn's and, in the face of the orthodoxy of medical opinion, was apparently dealing with it with diet and herbs. Whether I had Crohn's or not, Sophia was an inspiration to me. If she could do it, I could do it.

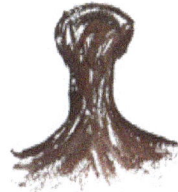

What Leila saw next

However, I was only thinking like this because I was afraid. It is fear that squeezes the heart and casts a sickly hue on the mind.

I didn't need the doctors to tell me something wasn't right. The whole silly saga was starting to spook me.

The eyes in the mirror were looking out at a world that looked familiar but wasn't, quite.

It was time to visit my seer again. Once more I made my way to Leila's quiet healing room in the regenerating Waiheke forest. Not without a touch of fear this time.

Leila's second reading did nothing to reduce that sense of strangeness – or the fear behind it. This time she did not see a pulsing point, but a dark, roughly circular shape with a root-like growth coming from it. 'It's growing,' she reported. 'The healing energies are very busy, but they can only try to contain it. They're putting a kind of containment around it.'

I thought of Fenris Wolf, that great rabid wolf of Norse Mythology who could not be killed so was chained in the bowels of the earth by the Assir, the Gods of Asgard. If Fenris were to get loose, the final war that would end the world, Ragnarok, would ensue.

But there was more than this. There was an image of a little

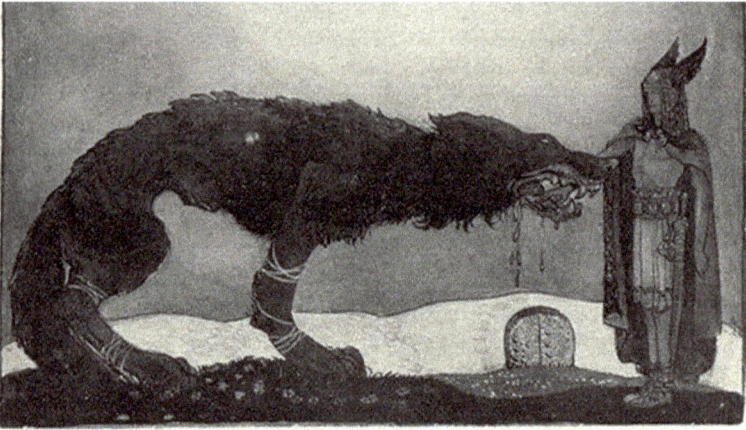

Tyr und Fenrir.

Fenris Wolf

boy in a very big lonely place. A little boy in a vast landscape. And Leila was called on to help this little boy, to begin the process of bringing him out of that lonely place. She didn't know what she was looking at but I had a fair idea.

Although I was born in Christchurch in 1947, my parents moved to Hanmer Springs, a tiny town on the edge of the Southern Alps when I was a few months old, and we lived there until I was five or six. Before I turned eight, we moved to Hinds, twelve-miles-south-of-Ashburton, as they said, and probably the loneliest place in Canterbury this side of the black stump.

After my last session with Leila, I was more convinced than ever that Janet was on the right track and we really did need to see what lay in those lonely painful reaches beyond the first bend, beyond the Sigmund.

I began to question my sense of well-being. Perhaps I was not as fit as I thought, how could I be? In the face of a creeping illness I might be compensating in my mind, pretending. A cognitive dissonance that opened the door to fear.

Janet came up with a plan. It was easier to get access to the CT scanner from within the hospital, as an in-patient, than from the outside, as an out-patient. This is the politics of health, the battle of the waiting lists. I imagine that all over town doctors are doing battle with hospital registrars to jump their patients up the list, or conniving to get them into hospital on some pretext so they can then jump all those out-patient jumpers.

I think it would have suited us better if I had been sicker. As Janet said as we finalised our plans – 'this is not the time to make light of your symptoms.' Of course, I understood.

So it was that on the morning of Monday, September 17th 2013, I entered Auckland hospital through the Accident and Emergency department.

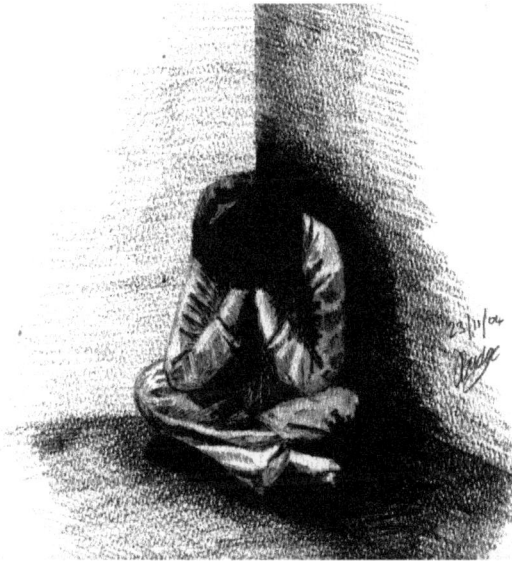

Loneliness – it goes with the territory.

September 17th, 2.21pm. Text to a friend:
It is very noisy and there are sick people everywhere.
I just want to have my tests and split.

It is clear from the email Janet sent me on Friday 14th that she envisaged a mere 'few days' for a CT scan and 'more blood tests etc.'

As it was, I would be in for nine days and would never be the same again.

I don't remember much about those first couple of days in Auckland hospital. The first thing you have to get used to is that, when you enter hospital, you enter a timeless temperature controlled zone in which the sense of day and night becomes slowly obliterated. I am sure it must be the same in prisons and factories of various kinds, especially those that must run 24/7 as they say.

This obliteration of our awareness of the 24-hour cycle might be counted by some as one of the triumphs of our industrial civilisation – another step towards freeing mankind from the tyranny of nature, another step forward in the mechanisation of society. Human consciousness is so malleable, isn't it?

For one thing there is no dark. I have heard there are people from the huge conurbations of Asia who have no experience of the dark, and find it hard to credit. Pollution makes their day into a gloomy brown, while at night bright lights pierce that gloom. What is day, what is night? I have heard that tourists come from these places to New Zealand just to experience night, and see, sometimes for the first time in their lives, the great canopy of stars we call the Milky Way. It's all so sad.

The next thing I noticed was the constant activity, patients in, patients out, visitors, medical personnel, orderlies, cleaners – there is a huge machine here to be served. Nor is there any sustained sleep. The hospital is a place where there is constant interruption, nurses coming in to test your vital functions (blood pressure, temperature, pulse rate, and/or take a blood sample) not to mention intermittent visits by doctors.

You might call it a controlled rumpus.

In such a situation it is difficult to sustain a sense of narrative, a sense of chronology, but from my text message record it's clear that the next day, Tuesday, I was moved from A & E whose admissions and planning ward is horrendously busy, to Ward 61 dubbed Elective Surgery, but was a hodgepodge of different cases – most waiting for tests or operations.

I was soon told to be prepared, that ninety-five percent of the time spent in hospital is spent waiting. Waiting for tests. Waiting for results. Waiting for procedures. Waiting to die. Waiting for time to resume its course.

So here I was, Ward 61, Room 4, Bed B. There was a reading light I could control and a button to summon the nurse. There was a cabinet with a deep narrow drawer on one side and a tray on the other. There was a cupboard just outside Room 4 where I could find sheets and pillowcases, and a kitchen around the corner for patients and visitors. There was a TV room beside the kitchen.

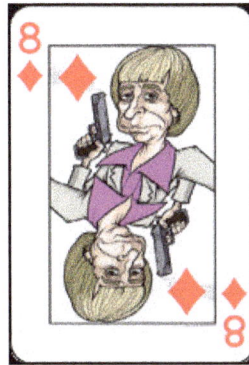

They don't call it escapism for nothing, honeykins

My move towards Ward 61 was somewhat of a mixed sign. It was welcome in one respect, that Ward 61 was somewhat quieter and more orderly than A & E, but it seemed to signal a longer stay than I anticipated. A sense of semi-permanence hung over one or two of the inmates, as if they had wandered in on their way home, never to find their way out. One of these was a skinny old Chinese man who sat in a chair by the one common window – a tall narrow window right at the end of the corridor – that offered a view of the eastern segment of the city and distant Rangitoto Island. He never did anything. He just sat and stared for hours on end, his face a mask. I imagined profound thoughts might be passing through his mind as he sat there in his pyjamas hardly moving a muscle, but then again maybe there was nothing at all passing through his mind. Nobody home, as the saying goes.

To begin with I think I treated it as a kind of holiday. I arrived at A & E lugging a pile of John Connelly's books, featuring his great middle-aged, angst-ridden detective, Hieronymus Bosch, as good a name for a fictional character as you are ever going to get. Bosch suited me just fine. He was an outstanding example of his kind, his genre, well graphed by Ian Rankin, and brought to a certain melancholy perfection by Henning Mankell in the form of Detective Kurt Wallanger. Like all of his kind, Bosch becomes obsessed with his cases; all the reader needs to do is hop on board.

Best of all Bosch's world of LA had nothing to do with Auckland Hospital, or a man in his sixties sitting up on a hospital bed thinking he's just taking a holiday and that soon this will, like some silly fiction in itself, all be over. That he'll pack up and go home and get on with his life. Just as Bosch will bring one case to a conclusion, nail a little of the vast evil in the world and get on with the next case. Bosch's world delivered me a card of quite a different kind.

All things considered, I was doing okay, and able to avoid most of the hospital food due to the support of my two wonderful daughters, Paloma and Sophia. I even managed to get out and take a walk in the park to keep my legs alive, as long as I kept my cellphone handy for instant recall to my hospital bed. It was not the done thing to be absent when a doctor paid a visit.

During that lone walk I could feel a familiar, reassuring surge of energy in my body, but at the same time I looked with envy on others enjoying the park. The white hospital band around my wrist didn't just identify, but marked me. I was in the world, like everybody else, but not of it.

I think of this time before the first CT scan, as the 'phoney war,' the calm before the storm. It almost seemed fitting that the weather outside was degenerating into a wet gusty gale, the cold variety that comes up from the south. Inside the hospital there is no weather, it's all temperature controlled, and while there is some comfort in being thus protected from the elements, the growing storm cut me off from the most important person in my life, Leila, my own wife and seer, an ocean away on Waiheke Island.

Tuesday evening arrived on long feathery legs, and loneliness was never far behind. I spent a lot of time with Bosch in his

---

My Doctors

1. Dr Head Honcho
Avuncular man with intelligent twinkling eyes. Great guy to have a yarn with – if you are not sitting in a hospital bed (two visits)
2. Dr Shiva and Dr Shanka
Dr Shiva was the nearest I had to a case doctor (three maybe four visits) His female offsider, Dr Shanka, was a late addition (two visits)
3. Ms Dr Immacula
One dramatic encounter, visited with Head Honcho once.
4. Young Male Doctor Number One *(two visits)*
5. Young Male Doctor Number Two *(one visit)*

Other Doctors
6. The First Colonoscopy Doctor
7. The No Nonsense Biopsy Doctor
8. The Second Colonoscopy Doctor

---

obsessive world. It was during this first halcyon period, waiting for the virtual colonoscopy, that I became an acute observer of hospital hierarchy and routine – at least its human aspect.

The alpha dogs are clearly the doctors who sweep around the corridors full of intent and purpose, often accompanied by an entourage made up of other less senior doctors, trainee doctors, students and other hangers on. A visit from 'The Doctor' is more like a visit from a delegation to your bedside. You lie on the bed looking the way you look while a group of faces peer interestedly at you. It's that alien abduction feeling again. It's hard to know in the old fashioned sense which doctor is your doctor or even if you have a dedicated doctor in that sense; the doctors can come from different departments or specialities. Then there are some doctors who never make a state visit to your bedside but into whose hands you are delivered for various procedures.

Below the doctors come the nurses, mostly women, and it is the nurses who are the heart and soul of the hospital. They do the day-to-day work of caring for patients. It is the nurses who work on the bleeding edge. Nurses tend to work three twelve-hour shifts followed by a three-day break, so you get to know your nurses better than anyone else. Staying on the friendly side of the nurses is an important tactical move for any patient. Because of their dominant role, nurses have more effective power than the doctors.

I can't mention nurses without thinking of Slither, as I rather unkindly came to call her in retrospect. She was there at the very beginning, and at the end, where she played her final part. She was the first nurse I had that first night in A & E. I might not have remembered her but that she shone a light in my face on that first night when I was trying to sleep and it made me feel like I was in prison.

'Don't shine the light in my face!' I hissed at her.

She said something like 'Just checking.'

Checking what? The question doesn't bear too close a scrutiny.

I didn't understand in those first couple of days that I had entered a new world, a world with many strange creatures in it, and that in this world there are those such as Slither, suddenly beside you with bloodtesting apparatus, or asking you if you needed paracetamol.

Below the nurses there are the student nurses, all young women, eager to do well in their practicum.

Below them there is quite a gulf to the orderlies, identifiable by their blue uniforms, taking the old laundry, filling up the cupboards with fresh laundry – and bringing around the meals. Special among these are those who wheeled you around from your ward to whatever department you might be called to for some test or other. These men seemed to me to be mostly late middle-aged Poms with bald heads and full of quips.

Below them are the cleaners and it was harder to get a handle on them, for they tend to cultivate invisibility. They are invariably women and they carry mops and they don't meet your eye. Most of them look like very tired immigrants with three jobs. These are the untouchables of the human hierarchy, yet I suspect they are at the front line in the battle against the hospital system's super-bugs, the dreaded antibiotic resistant killers that haunt the

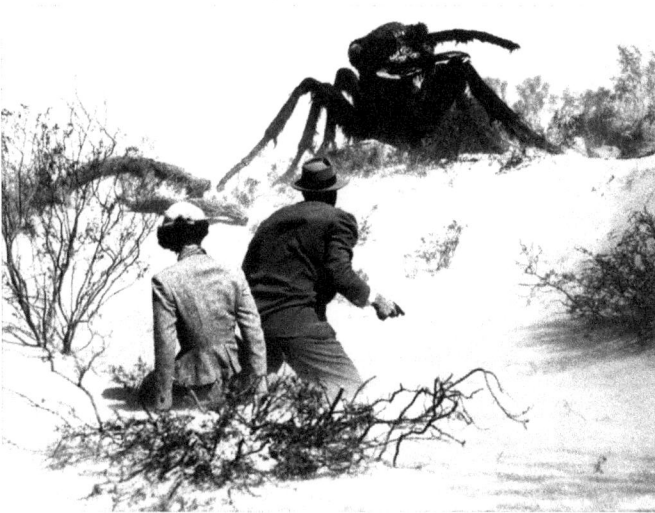

Having no natural predators, we have had to create our own.
Early prototypes show every sign of success.

corridors of modern medicine.

Everything has its shadow, its dark self, and for antibiotics it's the super-bug. The stronger one gets the stronger the other becomes. It is the paradox of medical power, and while it can't be banished, vigorous use of mop and disinfectant might hold the line for a little longer. In those hidden corners where the tired mop fails to reach, there death can bloom. How is it that a hospital, which should be a house of healing, is more often a place that breeds illness?

During those first few days of waiting and watching, I came to the attention of a student nurse I'm calling Felicity. She made a point of introducing herself when she was assigned to Room Four, and being friendly to each patient in turn. Her uniform announced she was from a local tertiary institution. She explained that she was on a three-week practicum and had been assigned to Ward 61. I was impressed by her calm intelligence and her steady grey eyes.

Later I was to ask her why she didn't choose to become a doctor and she replied, without a hint of reprimand, that being a nurse could be an intelligent choice too, and she preferred nursing because it was the nurses who were involved in direct care of the patients. Doctors, as she delicately put it, have a different job to do.

Feeling like a bit of a fool for the question, and the assumption that underlay it, I didn't help much by weakly commenting that she showed a wisdom beyond her years or some such rubbish.

'A lot of people have told me that,' she said sweetly.

A visit from the Head Honcho and his entourage confirmed that I would have the CT scan the following day, Wednesday. Leila was there for that visit, and did not form as favourable an impression of Head Honcho as I did. Then again, Leila has trouble with hospitals and doctors. The whole context of the place gets her fuming.

'This is not the way to heal people,' she says.

After the Head Honcho, had, like some visiting potentate,

made his grand exit, Leila settled in quietly to have a look at the bowel. I asked her to. Of course, the CT scan was a frightening prospect. I'd blocked the colonoscopy but there was no blocking x-rays. I was frightened of what they might find. Hospitals, as Leila has said, are not good places to do healings but there was no other choice. She simply sat quietly in the visitors' chair with her hands folded on her lap and her eyes closed. A casual observer might have thought she was praying. After some time she looked up, a bit puzzled.

'I can't see it,' she said.

'You mean Fenris wolf?'

'The growth I saw before, and all the containment. I can't see anything there at all now.'

But somehow neither of us felt lifted by the news. Maybe the hospital environment was interfering with her processes.

Tomorrow, the CT scan would tell the story.

3

The Night of the Blessing

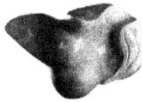

Excess of sorrow laughs
Excess of joy weeps
Joy impregnates
Sorrows bring forth.

William Blake, *Proverbs of Hell*

As all phoney wars must give way to the real thing and the fabled calm must give way before the storm, the Wednesday finally arrived, the day of the much-heralded CT scan, the virtual colonoscopy.

My God, I could have my scan and get out of there! Holiday over!

I had to fast for twelve hours before the scan, only take sips of water, but that was easy-peasy compared to drinking the gunk before a colonoscopy. The scan itself is even easier, as easy as getting an X-ray. All you have to do is lie on the rolling bed with a soft flexible X-ray plate over your 'tummy' and obey the little voice emanating from the machine saying, 'breathe in… breathe out…

…. stop breathing…'

At this point I undergo a time slip, or reality shift, or dislocation of memory, all of the above. I'm sitting on a hospital bed and I can't understand why I feel that someone has given me happy juice. Surely they don't give you drugs for a simple CT scan. A pretty Chinese woman is sitting beside me. It is Ms Dr Immacula but I don't remember her. There is some confusion. I've just asked her who she is, and it turns out she is a doctor and had visited me once before in the entourage of the Head Honcho. I find myself apologising for I'd taken her to be a student, whereas one look at her immaculate, snazzy black suit should have alerted me. This was, as Raymond Chandler might have put it, one fancy dame, far too young and immaculate to be a doctor.

I was finding it hard to concentrate on what she was telling me, what kind of language she was using. I looked around as if I'd never seen the room before, although I did recognise it. It was a waiting area or ante-room for the CT scan procedure room, I'd waited here before having the scan. Opposite me there was an alcoholic, florid-faced man sitting on the edge of a bed holding himself up by his arms. He didn't look too good. In fact he looked like he was about to die. Beside me was a very large Polynesian man lying on a bed.

He didn't look like he could sit up even if he wanted to. There was a desk by the door to the scanner room about which several nurses and student nurses clustered. They were smiling and laughing as if everything were normal.

I am slipping in and out of the present moment. Present and past and back to present again. Riding bareback, the future is at my shoulder.

Sitting beside me, on the end of my bed, is a pretty Chinese woman in a swish black dress and suit top. How small and delicate her face is! She is no more than a girl, surely. She is talking to me and I am trying to grasp the language. Primaries and metastases, lung, liver and bowel. I struggled to put it together. I looked at the man opposite. His face wasn't just florid it was mottled, purple and red, as were his arms and legs. Beside me the big Polynesian sighed.

'There is no sign of a primary in the bowel.' The Dr said. 'That's a good news.'

But she was talking about 'metastases,' on the liver and a 'secondary' in the lung... I can read back over the summary and report written later by Dr Shanka, and understand its deadly cool language, but I couldn't at that moment read Ms Dr Immacula's face, or the room. I didn't know why the group of nurses standing by the door were laughing or why a sterile grey light hung around everything in a sickly halo.

It came to me in fragments. This was cancer. She was talking about cancer, already quite advanced, it seemed.

On the liver.

In the lung.

She was assuring me that the CT scan failure to find a 'primary' did not mean there was no primary, just that they hadn't found it yet, and I would be kept over at the hospital pending a second CT scan whose dedicated purpose would be to survey the bowel to search for it.

From this I gathered that the scan I'd just had, the one before the time/memory split, had been more of a general survey. The second scan would get down to business: the Hunting of

---

The quest for certainty and the power of diagnosis.
The opposite of the placebo effect. Give them a harmless pill
and they feel better – point the bone and they die.

~

The expectation that death would result from having a bone pointed at a victim is not without foundation. Other similar rituals that cause death have been recorded around the world. (Wiki – Kurdaitcha)

~

Diagnosis, the primal power of naming. Give it a name and we know what it is – and how we might treat it. And often that works. But naming itself comes with fish-hooks, with ideological framing, with social loading, with judgement and emotion – and the illusion that by naming we control, have dominion over. It's all about authority. It's all about control.

the Snark. This is what it was really all about, this visit to the hospital under the pretext of doing a quick scan and getting out of there.

There was no getting out of there. Not now.

Then Ms Dr Immacula was gone.

I never saw her again.

The mottled man was still sitting opposite, propping himself up by his arms. The nurses were still clustered around the desk by the door. It was business as usual for them. I made some light-hearted remark for no particular reason. The big Polynesian man smiled as if he'd just met God.

And I was back in Ward 61, Room 4, Bed B, but there was no rest for me. Not that night. Maybe not ever again.

I was undergoing constant time/reality dislocations. You could say I was in a state of shock but that explains little. Memory, sliced and diced. Words cut out from people's mouths. Identity, a phantom to chase through the hours. One moment I would be sitting up in bed, trying to read of the adventures of Bosch who was no help here – this was way out of Detective Hieronymus Bosch's league: the case had taken a surprising and nasty twist. The next moment I would find myself walking the short corridors of Ward 61. Day had sliced into night. Outside, the storm blew big time, but when I stood beside the skinny Chinese guy in pyjamas and looked out, I couldn't see anything. Just smudged light and darkness. An impossible windy darkness.

The nurses took no notice of my restless movement – maybe they'd seen it all before.

I was on the phone to Leila. A voice that had to be mine was saying, 'There is very bad news behind the good news,' and Leila's voice, small and scared, from the other end of the universe, saying 'Yes, very bad news'.

At that moment when her tiny voice said that, I understood that, no matter how many reality shifts and time dislocations I went through, no matter through how many unlikely planes of

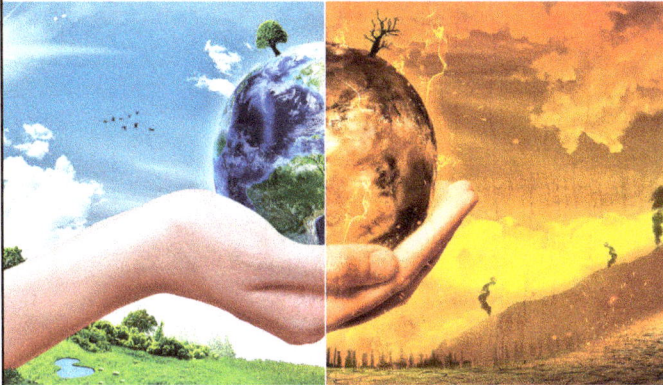

The Five Stages of Climate Change Denial

1. Deny the problem exists

2. a. Deny We are the cause

2. b. Consensus denial

3. Deny It is a problem

4. Deny We can solve it

5. It´s too Late (Self-fulfilling)

existence I passed, I would have to hold fast to the facts, no matter how unpalatable. The doors to the worlds of denial stood open and I couldn't go through one of them. I'd learned a lot about the mechanisms of denial by studying cultural reactions to the fact of human induced global warming. It was not superstition, or more rationality we needed – but a clear-headed facing of the evidence. A diagnosis had been made.

I was on the phone to Leila. I heard her voice say 'Very bad news' and I knew the bad news was my reality check. The bad news was all I had to hang onto. The bad news was my life-line.

The Five Stages of Cancer Denial

1. *The cancer doesn't exist. The experts have got it wrong again.*
2. *OK, it exists, but I am in no way responsible for my condition. All those years of boozing and abusing have nothing to do with it. It's an act of nature. And all those other boozers and abusers agree with me.*
3. *OK, it exists, but it's not really a problem. It's all part of God's plan. The experts will fix it. There might even be some side benefits. You don't have to die of cancer these days.*
4. *It's beyond solution. Nobody can solve it. There is no cure. I may as well just keep on boozing and abusing.*
5. *There may be solutions, cures, after all. But it's too late now! No use trying to close the door after the horse has bolted. I'm fucked!*

Everything else was la-di-da land, the land of false comforts and rationalisations. The little boy had arrived at the loneliest place.

I was walking the narrow paths of Ward 61, nothing more than an H shape really, with rooms on each side full of sick people – see, there's one of them now in Room 4, Bed B, sitting up in bed holding a book, a thriller, eyes unseeing like a blind man's. He's starting to get that hospital look about him.

I was going to die. It didn't really matter if it were six months or six years – sentence had been passed. I'd been lifted out of my old life and tossed onto a new one, a new path, and all I knew was that this path had only one destination. No stops along the way, no pausing to gather flowers from the fields adjoining. Once the path is joined there is no dilly-dallying – the Puritans had that much right. Straight is the gate, narrow is the way, and once the path is joined there is no looking right or left, no gainsaying the facts, no peering wistfully through open doors to illusory worlds and carrion comforts.

In their books on how to write stories, both Christopher Vogler and Robert McKee stress that the circle of narrative is a magic place insofar as everything within it, every object and action becomes charged, supercharged, with significance. In fiction there is no neutral ground. In real life, if that's what we call it, a glass of water might sit on the bench just because it's there, and carries no further burden. Not so in fiction. There is a glass of water on the table because the overall design of the story calls for it. It might fulfil its destiny by having poison slipped into it, or being tossed into a character's face. Our ordinary old glass of water requires no such destiny, no such justification.

As it is with objects, so it is with actions. According to Vogler, after successfully dealing with some threshold guardians, the magic world into which the character steps will be full of strange beings, shapeshifters, tricksters – friends, allies and enemies. People will not be what they seem. It is up to our protagonist to understand this new world into which he-she has been thrust, to understand it and master it! To control the forces it contains and use the laws it runs by to bring about the desired aim, whatever that may be. The rebalancing of the world!

What these writers on writing don't say is that the charged or supercharged nature of events is not limited to fiction. It can happen in real life, especially when real life suddenly gets a lot realer. In fact its fictional counterpart is probably only a pale reflection of the real thing, the crossing of the real threshold into an unknown land full of strangeness and terror.

The threshold guardians I had been grappling with during the period of reality shifts were nothing less than dread and terror – ah! There be dragons! Whenever the dread and terror got too much, reality would shift again and I would be lying in Bed B, Room 4 staring at the ceiling, or pacing the short halls of Ward 61, or standing by the window with the Chinese man in pyjamas waiting for time to resume its course.

I felt the full strangeness of the world I had entered. I was alert, but not paranoid. Just as the heroes of modern role-playing games might begin with or earn special powers and abilities so it

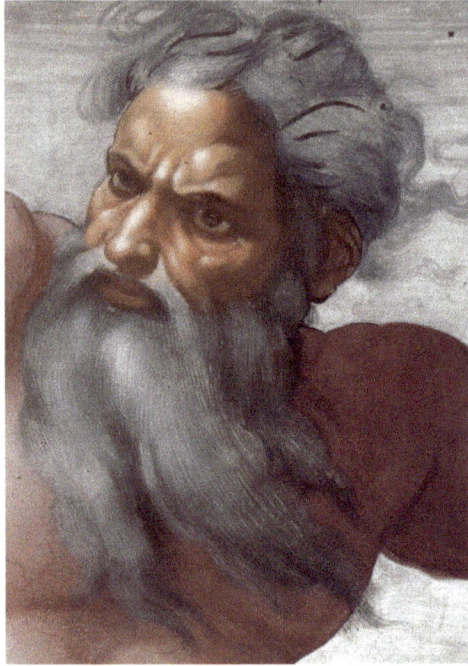

Son, this ain't a dream no more it's the real thing!

seemed with me. My helplessness and newness in this world were compensated by an enhanced clarity, a sharpness of perception. I could smell things from a distance, feel the hospital lean its concrete form into the wind. The enhanced clarity was a double-edged sword. On one hand I could cut through what I saw to its core, on the other, I could see myself still trapped in those time-shifts, those reality shifts, walking those same corridors, realising that the doors that provided access to Ward 61 were locked at night - at least, you could get out but you couldn't get back in, not without a swipe card and patients don't have swipe cards.

Silly, claustrophobic old man eyes wide shut in a daze, that's what the clarity revealed if I cared to look. Just as everything else in this world looked shabby. Even the light, some pale energy saver, drained the world of colour.

I had entered what the Christians might call the Dark Night of the Soul, and the concept takes us some distance. Where it doesn't take us is into that zone of absolute and irreversible change. That is the hallmark of this real life journey just as it is the hallmark of good fiction. Nothing will ever be the same again.

What qualifies it as a Dark Night of the Soul is the facing of death. The theoretical becomes the actual. The diagnosis had been made, the bone had been pointed, the battle joined. The double-edged sword was already in mid-air.

As Heidegger said in the 1930s, the dreadful has already happened.

Like me, readers have doubtless heard that a drowning person sees their whole life flashing before their eyes as they drown. I didn't experience any flashing – a little flashing might have been welcome – but I did see chunks of my life, mostly things I would prefer not to have to remember, passing before my eyes in a slow grind, as slow as my walking through the corridors of Ward 61. It was a sluggish and dreary grind indeed. Time would not resume its course. That grind of memory took place in some other space. I wasn't even there, I was just walking. Time would shift and split but the slow grind would continue, keeping its own time.

Chunks of narrative, quite tiny some of them, are flung clear from that dark night. I'm standing by the entrance to Room 4 looking in at the night nurses who occupy a central box. They don't look at me. They are busy working on computers. One of them leans back in her chair and deftly resets her ponytail. It's business as usual for her.

I am walking down the longest stretch of corridor the cramped conditions of Ward 61 allow, heading for the closed exit doors, when the student nurse Felicity approaches me.

'I'm not on your room tonight,' she says, 'but I'll come and see you if you like.'

'Oh you don't have to,' I said or something like that. It was hard to read her expression. There was a steady calmness about her. 'Actually,' I said, 'I've had some bad news.' Saying it back out loud like that for the first time since talking to Leila on the phone broke a spell. Another reality shift. I was back in real land. The exit door was closed. That was my own voice I heard in the real world. That was my own voice spelling it out back to me. Replaying it in real time, making it real over and over again.

I am sitting up in bed and Felicity is sitting beside me on a chair provided for visitors. We are talking, but I don't remember what about. Perhaps I kept trying to explain the whole thing, over and over, perhaps not. Perhaps I talk about my family, about Leila on Waiheke a storm and a world away. Perhaps I talk about my children, my eldest son also on Waiheke, my other son in Germany, my two daughters in Auckland. Even if I could, I wouldn't want to see them now, not in this place, and I don't mean the hospital. Or maybe we talked about none of these things. Maybe I talked about my job, about writing. I don't think I cried. I wouldn't want to. Crying in front of a strange young woman would fill me with shame. I found her presence both reassuring and disconcerting, as was her capacity for inner calm and steadiness of spirit.

Maybe it didn't matter what we talked about, until she said, absolutely unexpectedly, 'I think you need a hug.'

Every taboo in the book was against it. Student nurse. Lecturer. Out of sheer instinct I shied away.

'No, no, no that's not...' whatever I said.

More than anything I was frightened. I didn't understand any of this, not since that dislocated conversation with the mysterious Ms Dr Immaculata who, like the beautiful but wicked witch of fairy tale, had put a spell on me. A horrible spell. Now another young woman, also beautiful but in a much more earthy, ordinary way, was going to hug me. Would this lift Immaculata's spell?

'Yes, I'm going to hug you,' she announced. She was calm and quite firm about it. Tranquil almost.

And she did.

Without fear or embarrassment.

A blessing flowed through her body into mine.

The Dark Night of the Soul turned into the Night of the Blessing.

I didn't understand it, right there and then. What it was I had just experienced.

I didn't have a language for it, no precedent for it.

How can you comprehend or explain something that has never happened to you before?

'I have to go back to work now,' she said a few moments later.

Ten minutes later Leila rang. I was walking again. The short corridors.

'I saw an Angel of Compassion hovering over Auckland hospital,' Leila said. 'A very strong picture.'

Most of us have the wrong idea about angels. We think of cherubs with wings or Fin de Siècle, New-Agey apparitions of a Pre-Raphaelite, gauzy aspect. We have no conception of the sheer elemental power of such a living force, no clue of what

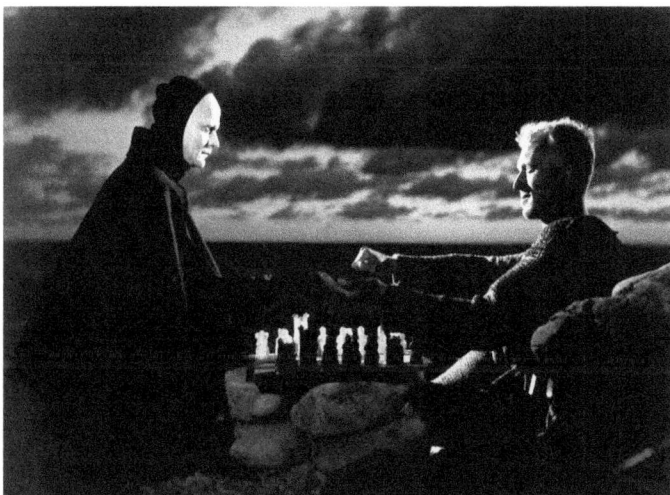

Your move!

Rilke might mean when he says that every angel brings terror, when he says that if one of them embraced him he would be consumed in that overwhelming existence.

If Leila had rung just a little earlier, I wouldn't have understood what she was talking about. I'd have seen a cherub floating in the sky. Even so I could barely grasp it; the magnitude of the gift had overwhelmed my ability to understand it. Leila had seen the Angel of Compassion somewhere around the moment Felicity hugged me.

Very dimly, like someone caught stupidly half awake, I understood that Rilke is talking quite literally. Unmediated, the raw energy of such a force would destroy us, consume us. Such a force is compassion, which is no less than unconditional love. To reach us without destroying us the angel force, if we can call it that, must work at one remove, through some agency which may not understand what is happening either.

In this case the student nurse Felicity was no Angel of Compassion, even if I could have turned her into a religion at the drop of a hat. She was just an ordinary young woman, smarter and more perceptive than many, but no ethereal being.

Compassion is the real force behind the Christian virtue of Charity, which some Christians characterise as a supernatural force, said to be the greatest of the virtues. Yet it is debased into a thoughtless coin into a cup. The word charity itself has come to imply its ironical opposite.

If I said I'd been on the receiving end of a young woman's charity, that would more than likely be misread, and not seen as the blessing that it was.

Leila was still on the phone. I was standing by the narrow window looking out at an endless storm. Waiheke Island was out there somewhere. I'm standing beside an empty chair. The Chinese man in pyjamas has gone. Leila is talking slowly and carefully. I think it has been a very short conversation. Just the message about the Angel of Compassion.

'There's more,' Leila is saying, 'Sometimes, in order to receive this kind of healing, you have to be... shifted... to another realm, you call them dimensions…'

'Do I?'

'It can be hard to return, to come back from that other realm. You can get lost there, stuck there, it's important to come back…'

Her voice rang in my ears. Come back! That's what I had to do. Already the blessing belonged to time. Felicity was just another student nurse in another room. I was standing by a narrow window holding a cellphone.

Come back! Come back! the cellphone is saying.

That's what I had to do.

Notes Towards a Theory of the Collapse of Opposites

The strict division we make between life and death, and the great fear this creates, may not stand scrutiny. So many times in the history of science and thought we have seen apparent opposites collapsed into one another.

Here are some examples:

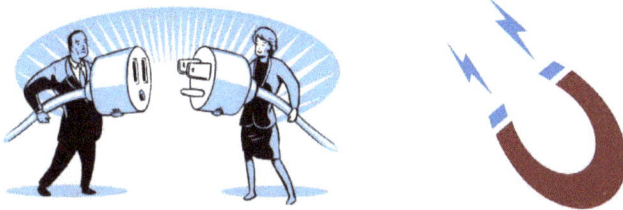

Electricity v Magnetism … electromagnetism. Seen as two separate forces, unified into one theory by James Maxwell, 1873.

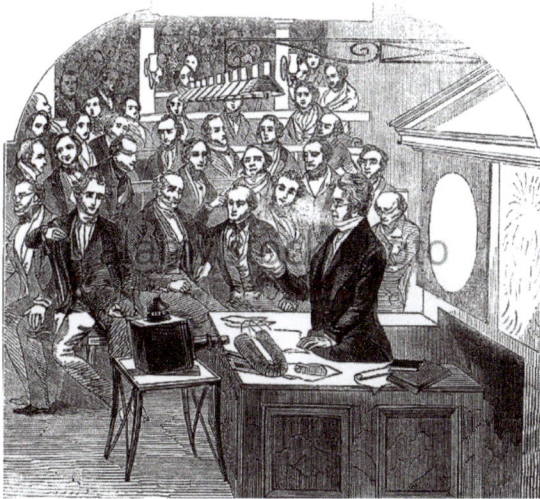

Michael Faraday lecturing on electricity and magnetism.

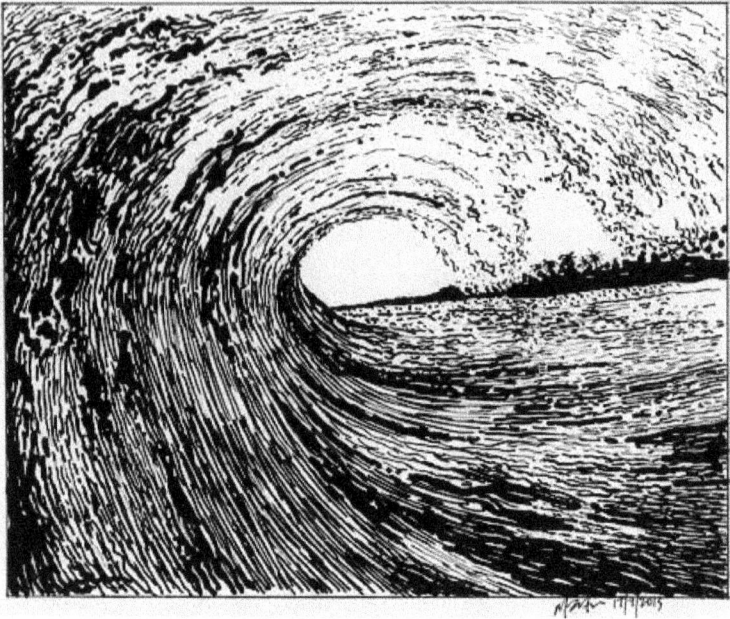

Matter v Energy ... e=mc2
Fundamental equivalence of matter and energy stated by Einstein
1905.

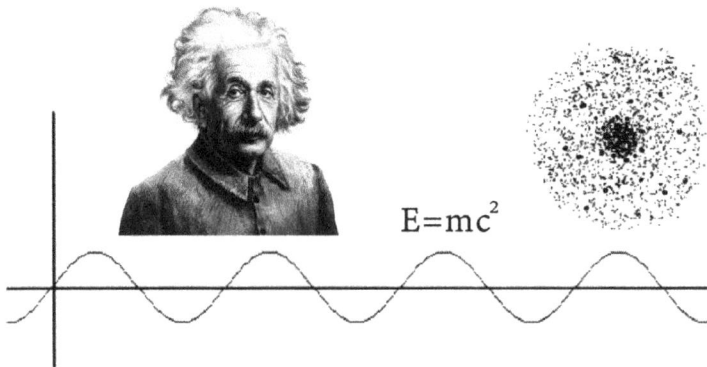

$$E=mc^2$$

The Double Slit Experiment

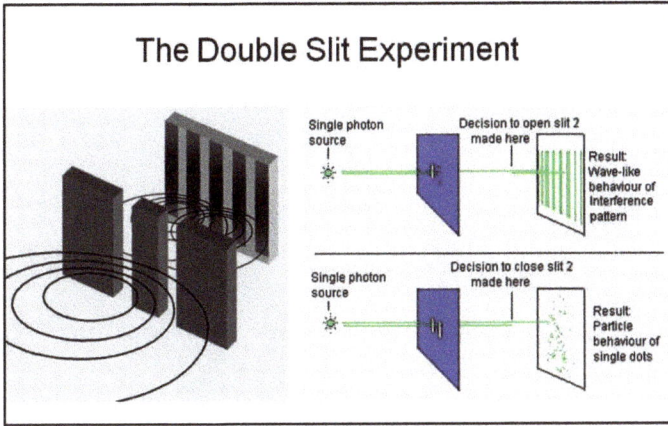

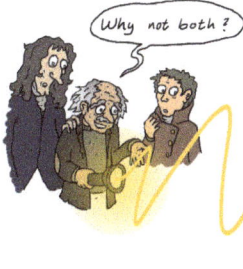

Particle v Wave … particle-wave. 1920s double slit experiment showed light could be measured as either a particle – photon – or wave front.

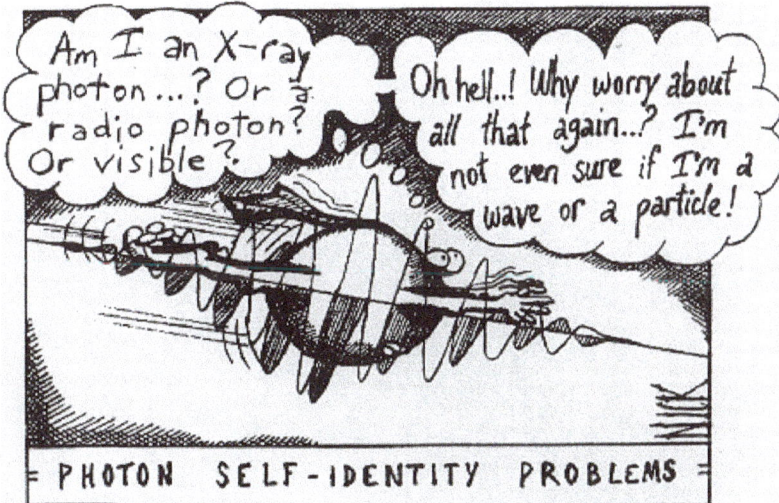

PHOTON SELF-IDENTITY PROBLEMS

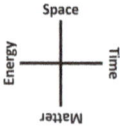

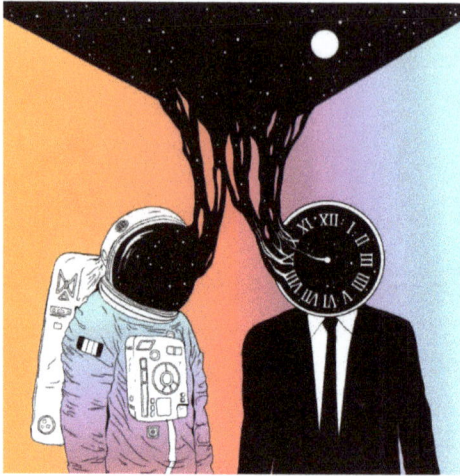

Space v Time … spacetime.
'There is no difference between time and any of the three dimensions
of space.' HG Wells, 1895. Maths supplied by Einstein, relativity
theory, 1905/1915.

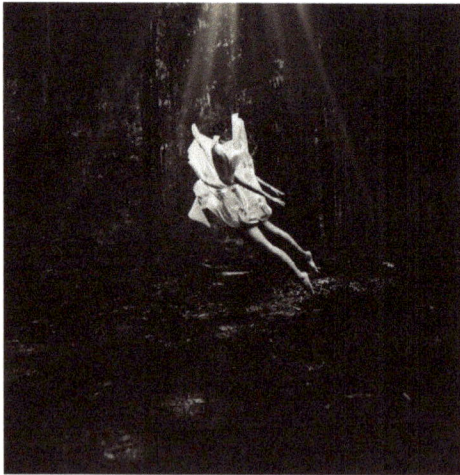

Cosmic Egg (Big Bang creation theory) v Steady State (continuous universe)… the multiverse.
Multiple big bangs within a stable, super-symmetrical 11 dimensional multiverse as delineated in M theory maths, an outgrowth of string theory, solves the cosmological argument.

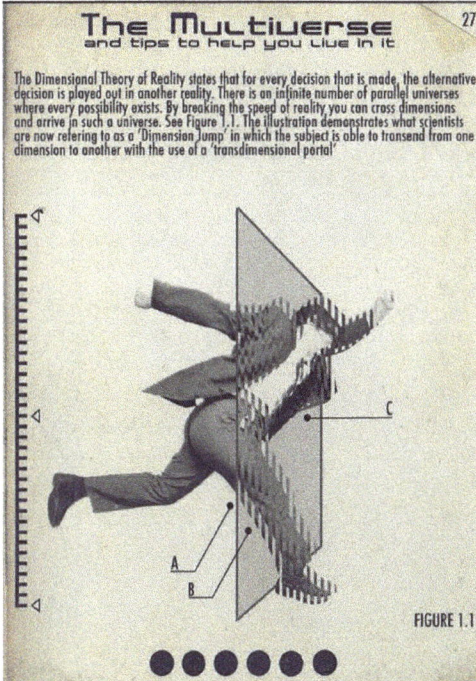

The Multiverse
and tips to help you live in it

The Dimensional Theory of Reality states that for every decision that is made, the alternative decision is played out in another reality. There is an infinite number of parallel universes where every possibility exists. By breaking the speed of reality you can cross dimensions and arrive in such a universe. See Figure 1.1. The illustration demonstrates what scientists are now refering to as a 'Dimension Jump' in which the subject is able to transcend from one dimension to another with the use of a 'transdimensional portal'

C
A
B
FIGURE 1.1

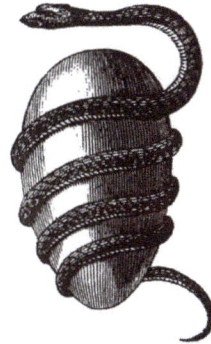

From Bryant's *An Analysis of Ancient Mythology.*

THE ORPHIC EGG.

The ancient symbol of the Orphic Myster-ies was the serpent-entwined egg, which signified Cosmos as encircled by the fiery Creative Spirit. The egg also represents the soul of the philosopher; the serpent, the Mysteries. At the time of initiation the shell is broken and man emerges from the embry-onic state of physical existence wherein he had remained through the fetal period of philosophic regeneration.

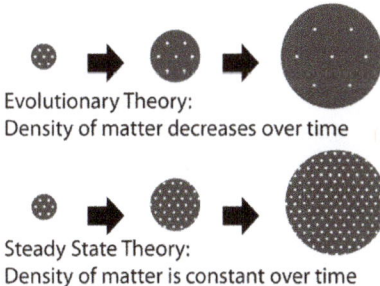

Evolutionary Theory:
Density of matter decreases over time

Steady State Theory:
Density of matter is constant over time

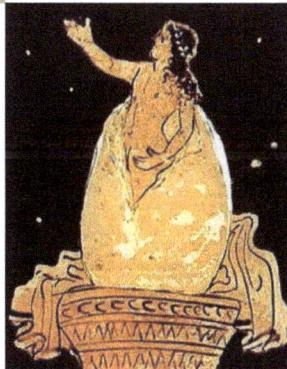

Angel of Compassion

It was like the abrupt dawn

Of a zillion stars

a ganglion of lightnings

for my consternation

Oh Lord of Dark Places

If you are light

There can be no metaphor

Darkness v Light ...
Allama Prabha (12th Century, India).

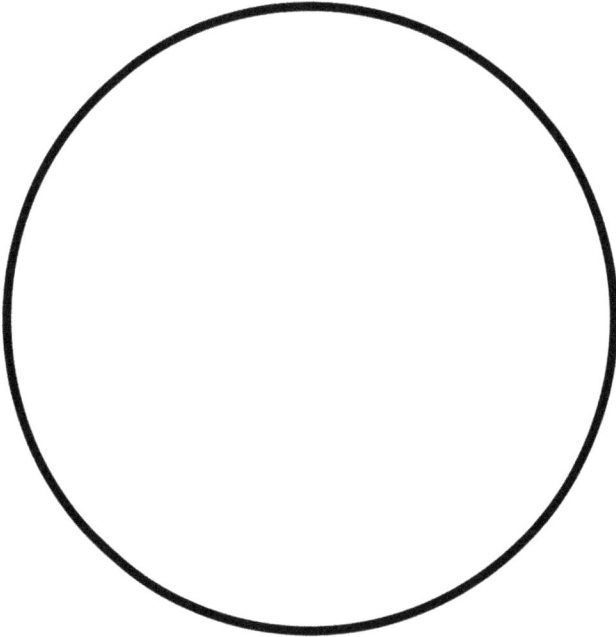

Life v Death

4

Scanners Darkly

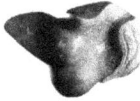

Run run as fast as you can
You can't catch me I'm the gingerbread man

It is not clear to what extent uncertainty underlies our relation to reality. Heisenberg's famous Uncertainty Principle is really a limited case, applying only to determining both position and momentum in a quantum world, in the particle zoo.

But that doesn't send the issue away. There are times when the nature of our uncertainties comes under scrutiny.

A diagnosis is a certain thing, a definitive answer – or is it? When is a diagnosis not a diagnosis? When the language changes.

With the CT Scan showing 'cancers', they were finally called cancers, on the liver, and suspicious activity on the lung, both assumed to be 'secondaries,' the hunt was on for the 'primary'. It was the Young Doctor Number One who told me the game plan. They were going to have a second attempt at a colonoscopy. And then, at the same time go in the other end, the mouth and down the gullet into the stomach with a camera – a procedure known as a gastroscopy. After that, on the same day, I would have a second CT scan.

He squatted down beside my bed as he told me this, the way you get down to a child's level so as not to appear to loom over them. It's probably in their training.

It didn't help. I didn't take the news well about the repeat colonoscopy, and questioned him about it. He said, in a rather roundabout way, that different 'operators' might get different results.

'Does that mean,' I said, 'that some doctors are better at it than others?'

He chose his words with great care. 'Not exactly. It means that the procedure is operator dependent.'

Operator dependent? Isn't that what I just said? This was getting tricky.

The language was growing shadows.

I agreed in the end, albeit reluctantly. I was in here for tests wasn't I? They sure were itching to get that camera up past the Sigmund. It was like starting all over again.

A Gastroscopy

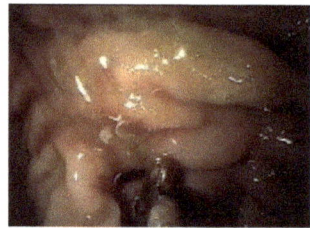

Another aspect of this bothered me. I was not as strong as I had been when I entered the hospital. The vital energy I had felt going for the walk in the park was fading. Fasting, a patchy diet, and the trauma of the diagnosis had leached away my body's strength and natural resilience. I was starting to get night fevers. Unexplained. My weight was dropping fast. Red blood cell count was dropping. Another period of fasting and force-clearing the bowel for a second colonoscopy would be a further body blow.

I was going downhill.

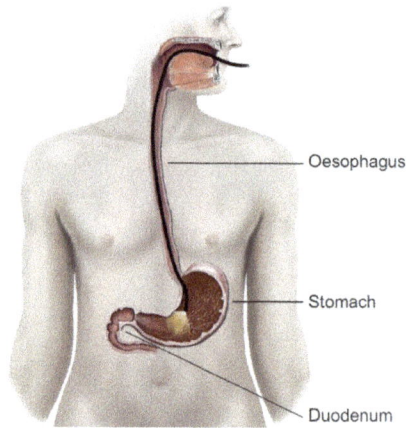

I was dying. Get out, come back!

But I agreed anyway. In for a penny in for a pound.

I wasn't feeling so great the next day. I wanted it all to be over so I could eat. I wanted to go for a walk in the park, a whistle in the dark. I wanted to feel the air on my face. I felt like a bleached pole. I was dreading the approaching colonoscopy and resented having to be wheeled around corridors in my bed.

I was still able to walk wasn't I?

And what was this testiness anyway? I'd seen it on the faces of others being wheeled around on beds, the sense of hopelessness and resignation and suppressed anger – a consequence of enforced passivity, being wheeled here, poked and prodded there. I saw the face of a bitter man and did not want to become him.

I was prepped and drugged in the now familiar fashion and rolled into the procedure room. There were two nurses, and a woman sitting at a computer. She was looking at a picture on the screen of a bowel, doubtless my own. The first scan had done a pretty good job of mapping it. Impressive technology; expensive too no doubt.

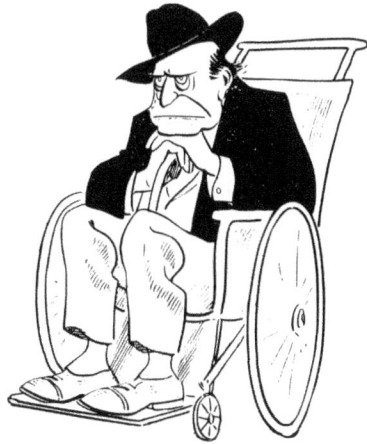

The two nurses I'd never seen before fussed around me, doing what they had to do. Nothing happened. The woman kept staring at the screen.

The nurses fussed some more and then fell quiet.

Nothing happened. Life went on around us.

Still nothing happened.

The woman swung around. I can't be sure that she was the same doctor I was later to call the no-nonsense woman, or Dr No-Nonsense; I wasn't observing clearly.

'I'm not doing it,' she said.

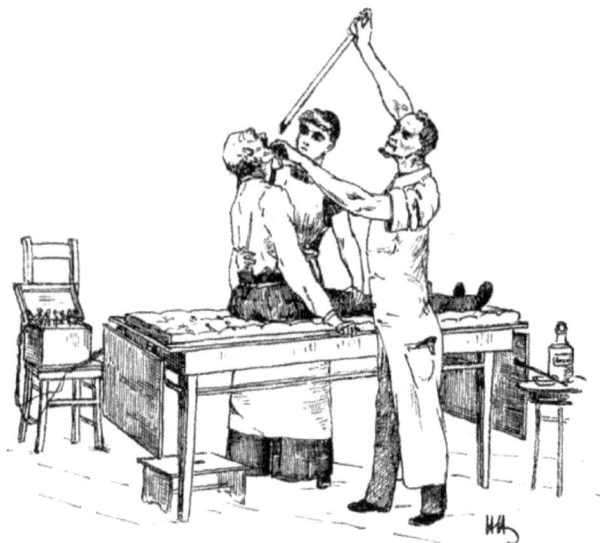

The nurses went very quiet.

'It's too dangerous,' she said. 'If we penetrate the bowel wall we'll have real problems.'

I had to agree with her. I hardly spared a thought for all that wasted gunk!

The gastroscopy was so easy, I don't remember it. Something went down my mouth and into my stomach. I remember ending up back in Room 4, Bed B, Ward 61, able to eat some real food and claw back some strength. They had cancelled the afternoon CT scan. More delay, but they managed to fit in a chest X-ray along the way.

The results came back the next morning. I think it was Dr Shiva. The gastroscopy had revealed nothing irregular in my stomach. And the chest X-ray found no offence in the lungs.

He spoke in a roundabout way. I wasn't sure what I was hearing. No metastases on the lung! So what had the first CT scan seen? Later he was to describe the lung phenomenon as 'nodules', a far more neutral term than cancers or metastases, but his language was already becoming more guarded. It was not clear what was happening in the lungs. I began to understand the power of naming. Language on the move again. I was pleased, yes, but bewildered too. If cancers could disappear from the lung maybe they could disappear from the liver too. What was the status of the images on the screen? Did the chest X-ray somehow trump the CT scan? That was hard to imagine, given the fancy scanner.

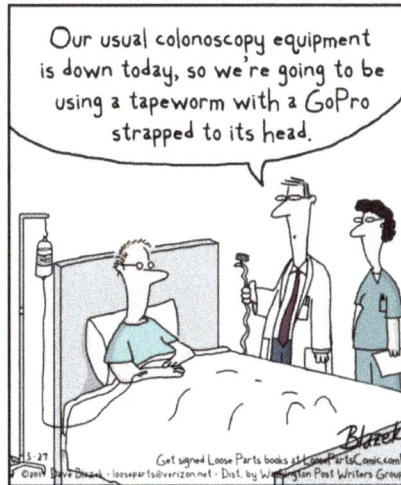

The next CT scan, which was now being called a virtual colonoscopy, was re-scheduled for the following day in the afternoon.

I tried to concentrate on other things, like reading my endless supply of John Connelly books, but the escapist thing wasn't quite working for me. No longer did the corrupt appearances-versus-reality world of LA seem so distant. Motifs began to leak from Bosch's universe into mine.

The murder book is a good example. Detective Hieronymus Bosch likes to carry around a ring binder in which all the interviews, reports and evidence relating to a case are collected chronologically. On reaching an impasse in a murder case, there was nothing Bosch relishes more than sitting down with the murder book, looking for clues, pointers that everybody has missed. The hidden key to the case. It's always there in the murder book, if you look hard enough. But Bosch's was not the only ring binder in my life. I began to notice that when doctors, and nurses starting a new shift, visited me, they carried just such a ring binder, with my name in large lettering on the side in blue marker ink. I imagined, not unreasonably, a growing pile of paperwork, a chronology, the dates and results of tests, what my vital signs were on the Night of the Blessing. It would all be in there. I imagined sitting with

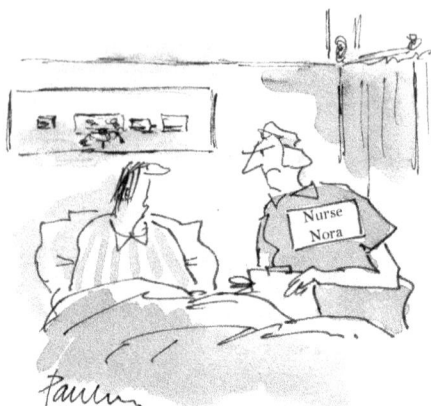

"Trust me, I'm a writer. My chart definitely needs more exclamation points."

Yesterday, upon the stair,
I met a man who wasn't there.
He wasn't there again today,
I wish, I wish he'd go away...

Hughes Mearns

it in front of me, staring at it in the way that Bosch stared at his murder book, searching for the elusive clue, the forgotten detail, the minor note that would bring the whole ensemble into harmony – the secret to my existence, my life and my death. A full picture of the evidence against me.

My medical record was starting to look suspiciously like Bosch's murder book. All the evidence was there. Other elements of Bosch's world would also leak through to mine. Bosch's world was full of the uncertainty of waiting. What you thought you saw wasn't what you saw. Here's a blind alley. Here's a false lead. Here's a clue overlooked.

The time for the virtual colonoscopy rolled around after more

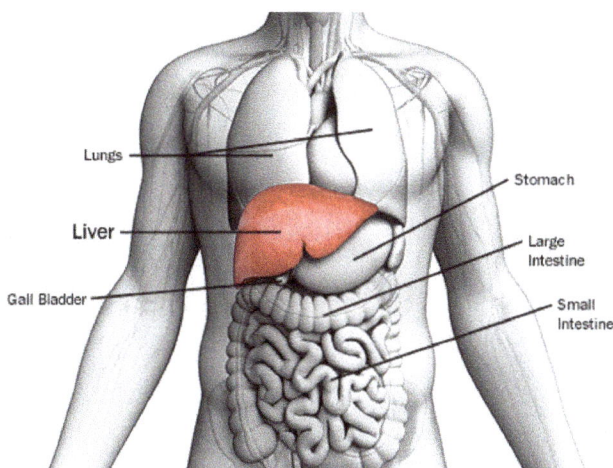

fasting. I was used to CT scans by now. An old hand in fact. 'Breathe in... stop breathing... breathe naturally...'

Exciting things were happening. I could leave the hospital in the morning, Saturday, return to Waiheke as long as I was back in hospital by Sunday 1pm. I was to be released on good behaviour! Home! Before returning to Waiheke I received the report from the virtual colonoscopy.

No traces of a cancer primary could be found.

There were the usual strictures. Just because they couldn't find a primary didn't mean there wasn't one. Don't forget these secondaries on the liver.

'Then it might be too small to see.'

Dr Shiva was reluctant to agree. He was thinking like a lawyer which got me thinking the same way. Leila's insights aside, the medical profession's idea that there was a primary in the bowel was nothing more than an assumption, not a diagnosis at all. A reasonable assumption, yes, but an assumption nevertheless. Presented to me however as a diagnosis in the process of being confirmed. It could be a false lead. Now doubts appeared to be setting in all around. The assumption that there must be a primary was behind their description of lung spots and liver spots as metastases. These were assumed to be colonies. Without the primary, how could there be any secondaries?

With the downgrading of the metastases in the lung to nodules, all that was left were the liver cancers.

'When you return from Waiheke we will do a biopsy,' Dr Shiva said with some confidence.

A liver biopsy, I learned, was a procedure in which a slender needle is inserted through the skin and guided to the cancers on the liver using an ultrasound camera. A sample is extracted. They can tell a lot by looking at those cells. Where they come from, for example, and the nature of their malignancy.

It was something to look forward to.

My Saturday trip to Waiheke is a red letter day in my mind, not just the release of being out of Ward 61 for a while, but because it is the last time I can remember, as I write this now, when I still had most of my old strength and energy.

My daughters swung into action. Sophia waited outside the hospital in the car while Paloma came up to Ward 61 to fetch me. I was concerned the sea would be rough after the storm, feeling very unready to face motion sickness. Paloma accompanied me on the ferry and I was glad for the company. It seemed like a very long time had passed since I had been on that ferry.

Leila was working that weekend, and the first thing I did when I got home was cook up a feast of fish, kumara, greens, herbs and whatever else I could find in the Paleo diet line. I finished it all up and I was still hungry. I was like the

> *it was*
> *as if the fire in the tree*
> *burned the tree*
>
> *as if the sweet smells*
> *of the winds of space*
> *took over the nostrils*
>
> *as if the doll of wax*
> *went up in flames*
>
> *I worshipped the Lord*
> *and lost the world.*

little hungry caterpillar of that book for toddlers – I couldn't get enough.

While a second lot was cooking Sophia rang up.

'Go for a walk,' she said.

I obeyed, turned off the meal and went walking. I walked a good distance but my legs were still hungry. My legs and my stomach both. I walked another good distance. Strength, flowing through my body! The wind, flowing through my body, clouds ripping up the sky. Everything was possible; nothing was possible. Energy jolted from the earth up through my feet.

Waiheke was looking wild and windswept after the storm but looked all the better for that. Like the ocean itself, an island has many moods, and some of its rougher moments I liked the best. It felt like I could drink the wind. I would have walked further but stomach hunger was back at me again, and I had the return journey to make.

Home, I packed away a second big meal and was still hungry.

Leila arrived and I made a maca powder drink thick with coconut cream and superfood sprinkled on top. We settled into domestic bliss. The smallest things delighted me. I greeted the dark and the stars like old friends.

When I returned to the hospital on Sunday as agreed, I had no idea I would go downhill so quickly.

I felt okay when I arrived. Paloma had accompanied me back on the ferry to Auckland where Sophia was waiting with her car. Both accompanied me back up to Ward 61. I wanted to give them something, so I sat on the bed and read them some poems from the little volume, *Speaking of Shiva*, a favourite collection. When Allama Prabhu calls for those who have 'roasted the kernals of the heart,' I think I understood.

After my daughters left, it was back to hospital realities again. Bad news continued to flow. My blood pressure was all over the place, red blood cell count still dropping, weight still dropping. I was nothing but skin and bone. Worst of all, my temperature was on the rise, and the night fever was getting worse. The Sunday night nurse insisted that I take some paracetamol.

On Monday Felicity approached and asked if she could write up my case for her student assessment. I understood she had to do a case study. I agreed readily enough. She was able to show me the 'murder book' which I understood I was not permitted to read and ponder. She showed me how my temperature, when spiking, entered a different colour band, like emergency codes, triggering certain responses such as offers of paracetamol to bring down the fever and increased monitoring of my vital signs – every two hours through the night instead of every four hours.

Fevers indicate infections and the hospital is very alert to infections, as well it might be.

I was intrigued that I didn't have, weren't allowed, it seems, direct access to the 'murder book'. It had my name on the side. It was a dossier on me. Like the police in a Bosch novel, the medical profession was building a case, but at present it was circumstantial. They lacked hard evidence, and the biopsy would provide that. Not just images on a screen but real cells to look at with electron microscopes.

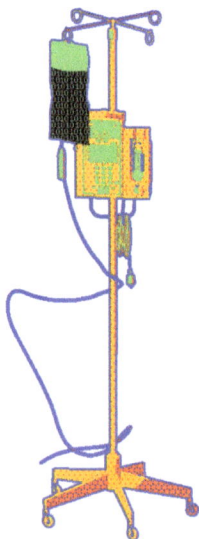

They took their time. I wasn't to go in for the biopsy until Wednesday midday. I wondered why I had to stay for two full days, days I could have spent on Waiheke. The answer was, if I stayed away I would lose my hospital bed, and so lose my place in the CT scan queue. To have the scan I had to stay hospitalised.

On Tuesday afternoon they put me on the drip and it was back to no food. The final fast I thought. The final assault, then I can go home for good. I had read eight John Connelly novels. The world of LA crime was wearing thin. It was time to go home.

The drip. That life saver. We didn't see it until afterwards. That saline solution

**Check with your doctor immediately if any of the
following side effects occur while taking quinine:**

More common
- *diarrhea*
- *nausea*
- *stomach cramps or pain*
- *vomiting*

Less common
- *anxiety*
- *behavior change, similar to drunkenness*
- *black, tarry stools*
- *blood in the urine or stools*
- *blurred vision or change in vision*
- *cold sweats*
- *confusion*
- *convulsions (seizures) or coma*
- *cool pale skin*
- *cough or hoarseness*
- *difficulty concentrating*
- *drowsiness*
- *excessive hunger*
- *fast heartbeat*
- *fever or chills*
- *headache*
- *lower back or side pain*
- *nervousness*
- *nightmares*
- *painful or difficult urination*
- *pinpoint red spots on the skin*
- *restless sleep*
- *shakiness*
- *slurred speech*
- *sore throat*
- *unusual bleeding or bruising*
- *unusual tiredness or weakness*

Rare
- *difficulty breathing or swallowing*
- *disturbed color perception*
- *double vision*
- *hives*
- *increased sweating*
- *muscle aches*
- *night blindness*
- *reddening of the skin, especially around ears*
- *ringing or buzzing in the ears*
- *swelling of the eyes, face, or inside of the nose*

contains sugar. Sugar acts as an accelerant on inflammatory bowel disease or irritable bowel syndrome. We'd been through that with Sophia. Apparently modern nutrition does not acknowledge the impact of what passes through the bowel on inflammatory bowel disease. It doesn't acknowledge the role of sugar, even though infections feed on sugar. I was mainlining the stuff, with no other food to balance it.

Tuesday, the day before the biopsy, I spent waiting – waiting and reading and deteriorating. There was a look, a look I'd seen in the faces of the older patients wandering the corridors toting their drips, a look hard to characterise. Bleached hopes. A lethargic will. The impossibility of resignation. No longer just among them, I was becoming one of them; no longer a stranger passing through, after eight days I was a long-termer in Ward 61. In Room 4 alone I'd seen several patients come and go. One of them, apparently scheduled for complicated cancer surgery involving multiple organs, checked himself out after one day declaring, 'I've had enough of this bullshit! I've got a company to run!' He had a deeply lined face and the yellow pallor of a dying man. He replaced the blind poet who'd wrecked his arm playing arm wrestling. There was a woman I'd never seen before carrying a baby and anxiously pacing the short halls of Ward 61. I'd outgrown my time here.

On Tuesday night my temperature went up to over 39 degrees. I imagined the spike on colour charts provoking a code alert. The nurse brought me paracetamol but I quietly dumped them in favour of the codeine-laced variety I had stashed in my bag.

Ah! the lucidity of fever! At least once before I had suffered a fever. It was the time of the little boy in the lonely place. When I was five going on six, I had six weeks of dangerous fever later diagnosed as polio – polio fever. I cheated death by never developing the paralysis. They treated me for scarlet fever and gave me quinine, and the quinine tore my brain open like a tin can.

On Wednesday morning, the day of the biopsy, my daughter

Paloma came to be my support person. Leila was to come later in the day, to get me out.

We didn't have to wait long. Soon I was being wheeled down to radiology by an orderly I already knew, a fast quipping Pom who thought I might care about a boat race happening in America. I was frightened again, like the proverbial rabbit in the headlights. Perhaps for just a moment the rabbit, frozen in time, doesn't believe the headlights are getting any bigger. You can fool around with images on a screen, but with a biopsy it's the real thing.

Felicity accompanied us on this mission, walking quietly beside us. She didn't appear to be listening to the conversation such as it was between me and Paloma, but I knew she was taking in every word. I think she was quite practiced at disguising her vigilance, her awareness. Since she was using me as a case study, she would be permitted to observe the procedure. It felt OK to have her there, but underneath it I was struggling to find the courage. Courage to get through the next few moments intact.

When we got to radiology I was parked next to the procedure room and, after the usual checklist of questions – double-check my identity – we were approached by a woman I immediately recognised as one of those highly competent, no-nonsense people, brisk if not brusque. Wiry and determined. I am sure she had a heavy workload. She introduced herself as the doctor who would perform the biopsy and quickly ascertained who Paloma and Felicity were. I asked her if Paloma might be permitted to come into the procedure room as a family support person.

'Absolutely not,' she replied. 'It's out of the question.'

A no-nonsense reply if ever I heard one. Without delay I was wheeled into the procedure room, Felicity beside me. There was an assistant nurse standing by a machine I knew to be an ultrasound, used to locate points of interest and guide the needle.

Cold gel was applied to my 'tummy' and I was instructed to lie on my back and my side in turn.

Dr No-Nonsense took the controls of the ultrasound. While the screen was not angled towards me for comfortable viewing,

I could, when lying on my back at least, catch a side-on view of the screen. It wasn't hard to see the liver. To my untrained eye it seemed as if the camera were orbiting some misshapen asteroid, pitted from a lifetime of meteor bombardment.

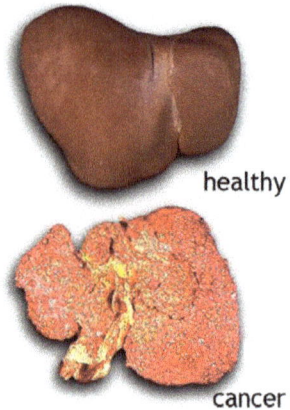

healthy

The camera continued to orbit and the asteroid continued to turn beneath our view. This went on for a while. The assistant nurse, who wore large glasses and had lots of teeth to smile, was quiet. Felicity was quiet.

cancer

When I rolled onto my side I couldn't see the screen but I could imagine it. I could feel the trace of the ultrasound receiver leaving a slug trail in the gel, the gel that was no longer cold, across my ribcage. It was heading for the other side, like the dark side of the moon. Then I had to roll on my back again.

'All I'm looking at is healthy liver tissue,' Dr No-Nonsense muttered, as if this were very much the sort of nonsense she could do without.

Five more minutes of orbiting the asteroid and we were already some fifteen minutes into what is booked as a half hour procedure.

'You'll have to excuse me for a moment,' she said. 'I can't find any lesions and have to check back on the CT scans.'

And she left the room.

While she was away, the assistant nurse, in the manner of an anxious but eager salesperson, assured me that Dr No-Nonsense was the most experienced and senior doctor in radiology and that the ultrasound was the very latest of equipment.

After five minutes she returned and resumed her place at the machine, once more quietly guiding the camera over my skin. At first she moved quite rapidly, with a sense of purpose. Then she slowed down and moved inch by inch over the territory below. Even I was starting to recognise some of the landmarks. We'd passed this way before. Five minutes went by. I could feel her frustration building. If she could see them on the CT scan why not now?

Finally she put the camera down.

'I can't complete the procedure because I can't find any lesions to biopsy,' she announced. She gestured for me to be wheeled out. My heart gave a tap dance.

'Excuse me,' I said. 'You've done lots of these procedures?'

She shrugged as if to indicate countless numbers. This was her job.

'How often does this happen, this failure to find the lesions?'

She looked at me then, actually focussed. Old fashioned writers would say, 'her eyes narrowed.' Not so much a suspicious look – after all, how could I be responsible – but a look nevertheless which said that if there was any nonsense going on here, she would soon ferret it out.

Medical sonography (ultrasonography) *is an ultrasound-based diagnostic medical imaging technique used to visualize muscles, tendons, and many internal organs, to capture their size, structure and any pathological lesions with real time tomographic images. Ultrasound has been used by radiologists and sonographers to image the human body for at least 50 years and has become a widely used diagnostic tool. The technology is relatively inexpensive and portable, especially when compared with other techniques, such as magnetic resonance imaging (MRI) and computed tomography (CT).*

Obscurely, I felt guilty as if it were my fault, that I had somehow been a naughty boy.

'Very, very rarely,' she said, and thought for a moment.

'In fact, the only case I can remember was a Polynesian man who was so large there was too much fat to see the liver. Never in anyone as skinny as you.'

And out she walked, the last time I saw her. The assisting nurse wheeled me out of the procedure room. She was no longer smiling.

'Well,' I said to Felicity, 'doesn't look like you have a typical case to write up.'

'That's right,' she said. Her face showed little. Her grey eyes remained calm and steady, which was not the way I was feeling. Something astonishing had happened but the world carried on as if everything were normal, at least the world of the hospital. Orderlies were wheeling patients to and fro. Nurses were hurrying purposefully about. The occasional doctor could be seen on obscure and important business. Just how astonishing this failed biopsy was we were to find out later, through a family contact who was the head supervising nurse in the oncology department. She, in all her twenty-five years' experience, had never heard of this happening. If it's on the scan it's there. The ultrasound is used to locate the exact spot for the biopsy.

The official status of these liver 'cancers', now called 'lesions' was that they were both there and not there. There on two CT scans, not there on the ultrasound.

Paloma was waiting for me outside the procedure room. We couldn't help gaping at each other with joy and bewilderment. No lesions! Felicity looked discretely down as Paloma and I hugged with joy. Somehow we had beaten the bastards, at least in the meantime. 'You know,' I said to Paloma in a burst of some kind of wild hope, 'I think Leila has been up to her tricks again.'

I was embarrassed because Felicity overheard me say that – she must have thought we were crazy – and in that moment we were crazy. In that moment I believed that Leila could do anything, even spirit cancers away from the liver! I was a believer. It could even be that the healing energies that Leila talks of, those energies, like compassion, that have the power to transform matter, were working through the unobtrusive presence of Felicity as they had already once done. I was suspicious of the coincidence of her being in the autopsy room. I was ready to see the hand of God, or at least the higher powers, in anything and everything, and couldn't rule out the possibility that the cancers had been there and had subsequently disappeared. That made just as much sense, or non-sense, as believing the cancers both did and didn't exist depending on the scanner you used.

Soon the orderly came to wheel us away. He wasn't a believer. It was all the same to him. Some would cry, some would laugh, some would just stare like zombies who had forgotten how to walk. All he had to do was push them around. Miracles in the autopsy room were way above his pay scale. I could have told him that the CT scanner was hallucinating and he wouldn't have turned a hair.

Felicity must have left us at the main desk of Ward 61 because she wasn't with us as I took up my old position in Berth B, Room 4. Leila was there, sitting quietly on a chair. She took one look at our faces. It was all she needed.

'What have you done!' Paloma said. She didn't shout. You don't shout in hospital – they are a bit like churches in that respect – but there was no containing the suppressed excitement of her voice.

'I didn't do anything,' Leila said and she buried her face in her hands as if she were guilty or having to hide away from the world, or maybe just from the hospital. 'I didn't do anything, just a little bit of liver support last night.'

Just a 'little bit' of liver support.

I had no way of assimilating or interpreting these events, and still don't. Later, more sober reflection was not able to throw the cooler light of reason on the autopsy room 'miracle' either. While it is generally recognised that the CT scan was more complete than ultrasound, able to build up three dimensional images of the scanned organs, the modern ultrasound was the equipment of choice for biopsies, and I had been able to find no record, at least via google, of any event like this taking place. I was a medical anomaly.

Shortly after that Dr Shiva arrived to make it official. To advise us that the biopsy had failed and that I could be discharged. To give him his due, he was looking quite uncomfortable. First he'd had to tell me that the lung cancers were polyps, now he had to bear the good news that the liver cancers had vanished.

After that there was a period of confusion as I got ready to leave the hospital. Leila was there at my elbow, getting me dressed and packing away the John Connelly novels. I had managed to read one novel for each day in hospital.

I needed help. My disorientation was profound, with roots deep in the challenge these events presented and the creeping fever that was now coming up on me. The cancers were like that sideshow trick with the pea and the three eggcups. Move the eggcups around fast enough and you'll never guess which one is hiding the pea. Now you see it now you don't. It's there but you can't see it when you look at it. Some readers might be of an age, or be cult movie freaks, and remember a late 1960's film by Antonioni called 'Blow Up'. It was quite a famous film in its day for its various daring scenes, but the story, what there was of it, revolved around the image of a gun that appeared in a photograph. However the weapon could only be seen at a certain magnification, the blow up. Magnify it further and the weapon disappeared in the miasma of shapes and colours. Make it smaller down to normal size and there was no gun in a man's hand. What is to be believed? Does the pistol exist or not? If it exists, why can it only be seen at a certain magnification; if it doesn't exist, how come it appears at all?

The film doesn't attempt to answer the questions – this was avant-garde land – but I was trying to answer mine. Through a Scanner Darkly, as Philip K. Dick put it.

It's just the fever, I thought. None of this is really happening. Everything seems lurid when you have a fever, a bit like tripping; you have to watch yourself.

We had to wait for Dr Kali to prepare the release form and a summary paper. This was only the second time we had met her. She had been with Dr Shiva the first time. Now we waited for her to complete the paper work.

That's when nurse Slither, my duty nurse for the day, made her move. Although I was dressed and ready to leave she would do her duty and take my vital signs one last time. Leila didn't want that to happen, but resignedly I let her take my temperature and blood pressure. My blood pressure was okay, but my temperature was over 38. I was oblivious somehow to Leila's agitation. I was trying to absorb this new information. I was running a fever, that was not my imagination. Slither was acting strangely, as if she knew something I didn't – like, for example, that I would have to stay in hospital and never get out – the 'Hotel California' syndrome. You can check out but you can't leave.

The frightening thing was, Leila said afterwards, that it seemed for a moment, as Slither made her play, that I somehow wanted to stay, couldn't rip myself loose. When Dr Kali finally gave us our release and our summary, Leila took me firmly by the hand and walked me down the exit corridor of Ward 61 for the last time. Felicity passed, going the other way. She gave us a quick look. Something had happened, she knew that. Something she didn't understand. Well, I didn't understand it either. All I knew was that I was being whisked down the lift and out into the cold, wet, blustery night in search of a taxi. Leila became more agitated as the taxi took its time. It felt to her as if the hospital were sucking me back in.

A Pommie Buddhist taxi driver took us down to the ferry. He was philosophical about looking like a Muslim. We had left but the hospital hadn't quite let go. Leila received a text from Dr Kali saying that I was running a temperature because of a flare-up of diverticulitis. A prescription would be faxed through to the Oneroa Chemist.

Leila acknowledged the text.

I was out, heading into the wet shiny dark. We were early for the ferry so I had some baked oysters at the wharf restaurant. It was starting to dawn on me. I was out. But where was I? I was out, but not out of the woods. The strangest events were yet to take place. The journey was not over. It would never be over.

⚠ **WARNING**

EXPOSED VOID
OPEN DOOR
WITH CARE

5

Fevre Dream

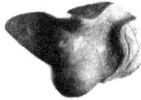

Does the road wind uphill all the way?
Yes to the very end.
Will the journey take the whole long day?
From morn till night my friend.

Christina Rossetti

In the days of the Old and the New Testaments, the prophets would induce fevers by fasting and refusing water and spending days in the hot sun of the deserts. They would bring about such a fevered state in order to 'see God' or commune with him, or have visions or whatever. Here, the body's chemistry is being used, manipulated even, as a means to an end, that end being determined by the overall intention. So what determines what, what causes what? You pays your money and you takes your chance. One thing begins to look certain. The Behaviourist notion, amazingly persistent as it offers a view of mankind as mechanism, which suits the world view of dominant interests, that we are nothing more than stimulus and response, cannot be sustained.
Besides these deeper questions of cause and effect, there is a puzzle just on the physical level itself. When Dr Kali texted Leila

Imagine for a moment the boiling and steaming mud pools from Rotorua. They are a nature picture for the action of our metabolism. In our metabolic system heat is produced and if the digestion is upset gas is produced similar to the sulphur smells of Rotorua. Imagine that this increased activity of the metabolic system starts to heat up the whole body, then you have a fever. One can say: Fever is a result of an increased metabolic activity. Fever is the most important help for our bodies to overcome many illnesses that challenge our health. Fever activates the immune system. It stops viruses and bacteria growing. The strengthening effect of fever seems to last a long time: One has found that patients who develop cancer have had very few feverish illnesses in their past, not even in their childhood.

Maybe you observed that a child gets ill after an overwhelming experience e.g. a visit of a family friend who lives far away. One can see here fever helps digest experiences. During a fever the whole organism goes through a 'smeltering' process which changes the body substance right into the protein structure.

Dr. Ulrich Doering

in the taxi on the way to the ferry, ascribing my temperature rise to a flare-up of diverticulitis, she was only guessing. The speculative nature of that diagnosis was later to be confirmed by Dr Shiva, who admitted that they did not know what caused the fever. When I first, those now two long months ago, went to see the doctor with abdominal pain, I had no temperature. When I came out of the hospital I was running a temperature but had no abdominal pain. My initial abdominal pain had been ascribed to diverticulitis. So, back on Waiheke, why wasn't I suffering abdominal pain? The origin of the fever remained a mystery.

It was possible that the fever was not an outcome of any illness the tests were meant to discover, but a nameless infection from the hospital, not quite a superbug but a bug nevertheless. The hospital's own contribution to my decline. Or it was there because it had to be there, because my inflammation markers were up. They were in fact so high it would be remarkable if I weren't

> *The primary tenet of behaviorism, as expressed in the writings of John B. Watson, B. F. Skinner, and others, is that psychology should concern itself with the observable behavior of people and animals, not with unobservable events that take place in their minds. The behaviorist school of thought maintains that behaviors as such can be described scientifically without recourse either to internal physiological events or to hypothetical constructs such as thoughts and beliefs.*

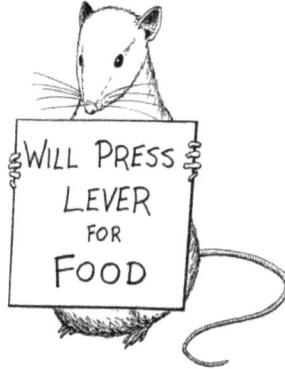

WILL PRESS
LEVER
FOR
FOOD

running a temperature. Or the question could be pushed in a different direction. Perhaps this was not a new or recent thing at all, this fever, that I had been harbouring it since that little boy lay on the hospital bed in Hanmer Springs sweating white beads. Perhaps the fever never left him, entirely, and was now let loose from the memory of the body.

In subsequent healings Leila found herself having to do a lot of work around the heart, where bacteria like to go to kill people. Leila has said that I came very close to dying in those first few days out of hospital, the closest moment I remember quite clearly.

Lacking anything other than a speculative diagnosis we had no way of knowing for sure. We were only making further assumptions, reasonable or unreasonable as they may be.

The fever would follow the same pattern every day. At first, for an hour or so after breakfast, it would hover from normal to the top of the normal range, between 36.8 and 37 degrees. Then as the afternoon set in, the temperature would slowly rise, 37.4, 37.6, 37.8. As it rose, my sense of crisis would deepen. I had many things to learn, to uncover and discover.

Besides, I was under orders.

Looks funny written that way, but that's the nearest I can get to the sensation. Everything I did was guided. *Drink water. Walk. Rest. Ring so-and-so and have a conversation about such and such. Remember this. Don't remember that. Start writing in the moleskin notebook Leila gave you. Eat this, don't eat that.*

How did I receive these instructions? Not voices exactly, more a kind of sudden knowledge. Such-and-such had to be done, there was nothing else to do but that. Call them compelling urges. I didn't just get an idea it might be nice to take off my shirt and sit in the hot spring morning sun, I had to do it.

As I say, I was under orders.

Leila knew this as some kind of sacred state; the healers had taken over and were guiding me, my every step, along the way. I was not so sure. As a teenager I read a remarkable book, one which made a lasting impression upon me. It was an account of schizophrenia, but to me it read like a science fiction story. One morning a young woman woke up to find several fuzzy figures standing around her bed, treating her as if they knew her well. These were her 'operators'. They would tell her what to do and where to go and how to manage her deteriorating psyche, which needed lots of repair. They told her which analyst to go to,

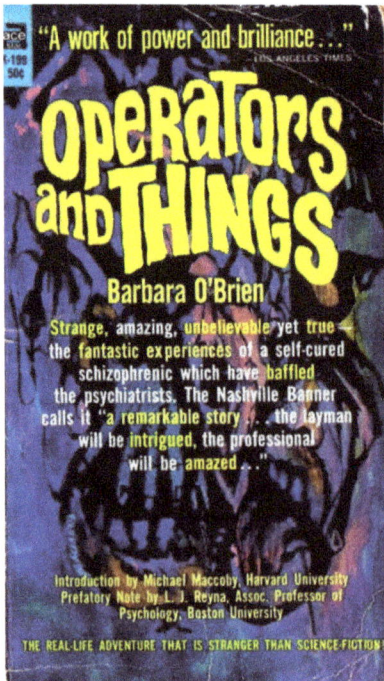

and which to avoid, whether or not to go to hospital etc. While their purpose was benign and made for a remarkable story, not all inner promptings, voices or materialisations are. Equally, the voice could tell you to go kill someone, and you'd do it because it would be the only thing to do.

Whatever qualms I might have had didn't make any difference. I was aware of a huge amount of internal activity, or activity on the etheric plane, to use Leila's language of the moment. I was no longer me, quasi-stable identity known to myself and others, I was a hive, a very busy place, where there was a lot of work to do. The activity grew so noisy Leila had to stop sleeping with me for a few days. On the last night she was awoken by a righteous old Scotsman who told her that this was no time for me to be 'fooling around with floozies.' She should take herself off as the laddie had work to do. One of my ancestors, apparently, keeping me on the straight and narrow.

So what kind of work were they talking about? Here the details get hazier. In one case I was part of a team working in Auckland Hospital, assiduously healing. I made some kind of breakthrough, an act of clarity which enabled others to do certain kinds of work, and that created a general sense of excitement and urgency among the etheric healers. Great urgency. I sensed these etheric others around me rather than saw them, yet sometimes a presence came close enough for me to almost but never quite hear it and see it. I felt the presence though, and it was a powerful one.

Just what this insight or clarity was I could never bring across from that world into this. These were the deep nights when the fever was at its maximum. The rules were those that applied to dreams. I didn't sleep – all that furious activity couldn't pass for sleep; and my fevered days could hardly pass for wakefulness.

But I wasn't always drawn back to the hospital, at least not Auckland Hospital, for there was another hospital that lay hidden, like a palimpsest beneath the remembered corridors of Ward 61, a hospital that lay deeper in my past. My work was to go back to that hospital and attend to the little boy there, the lonely little boy who was having a lot of trouble coming into the world – physical birth is only the beginning of a long process – and who was now lying on creased starchy white sheets in a hospital bed deep in fever, in polio fever, and was far from the world. 'Six weeks,' I kept hearing, 'he's been gone six weeks.' The number of years of his life. Gone. Gone where? Out of his body. He needs to come back. To come back into the world from wherever he has gone. I could see his skinny body curled in a foetal ball and wondered what could I do for him, me just a visiting spirit from Faraway.

I didn't understand what I was supposed to do. All I knew was that he and I are linked, linked through the fevre dream, a realm in which our times are joined, his and mine.

Because I don't know what to do, I remember. It is before the little boy got polio fever. He is standing outside the hospital under a sycamore tree, watching the seeds fall. Weighed at one end by the seed, it possesses only one wing, with a membrane like that of an insect, and has an unusual fluttery off-balance motion which, in a breeze, can whirl it quite a distance from the tree. The little boy watches the seeds fall. He is fascinated, as he is by the dark underside of snowflakes drifting down from the sky

The little boy is standing outside his parents' room. It is cold and damp in the house but he doesn't care. He only cares about the terrors that come to him at night, and have been coming every night since his fever. The fever has passed on but the terror is still there. He waits in silence, barely daring to move or even breathe until he is certain that his parents are asleep. He won't be confident of that until he can hear them snoring. His father, deep and uneven. His mother, light and steady. The dark of the house breeds shadows, but he ignores them. He concentrates on the waiting, the listening, the sound of his parents breathing. When he is certain they are asleep, he slips into bed on his mother's side, like a shadow. If he is lucky she won't wake up and question him. In the shared warmth, he will be able to sleep.

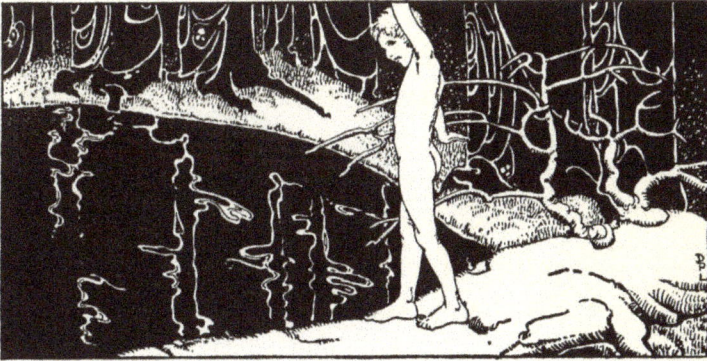

in winter, rotating each on its own axis. But the sycamore seed has no apparent axis. It has a lopsided, elliptical motion the boy likes. He watches the seeds fall, or the same seed fall over and over again in his fevre dream. Above him the sycamore spreads its cool branches. The little boy likes the tree and its circus seeds. And the tree likes him. Such trees love to amuse children with the comedy of their devices. Besides, trees root deep in the sky and flower deep in the earth. They are here. They are not lost. They have nowhere to come back from.

I revisited this territory several times. During that time Leila did a healing and perceived a being who spoke to me. He talked to me about images, how my mind worked with images. Then came the bombshell.

'The quinine you were given as a child force stripped images from your mind. And there was damage.' Pause. 'Now you must unpeel these fused images.'

In some manner the fever enabled me to do that. A process of uncovering, unmasking, and in many cases seeing these things was enough to change them, if only fractionally. I did some research too and began to doubt the diagnosis of polio fever for the little boy lost between realms, I was starting to doubt the source of my own fever as diverticulitis.

> *The signs and symbols of the world are there to be read. Once, while walking up our path to the house, I caught an odd movement out of the corner of my eye. It was a worm, a single long thread no thicker than a hair, pure white, moving blindly in a series of convoluted twists and undulations. It was blind, but it sensed its way forward by lifting a segment of what became its front into the air and waving about in a peculiarly graceful motion. Although I have lived in this valley for thirty years I have never seen such a creature. The point about it is that it does not need explaining, nor should it be reduced to some symbolic meaning which is then explicated, analysed and catalogued. This real life dream creature speaks to us in being what it is. Like the language of dreams.*

I couldn't find any account of the progression of polio that matched what I'd been told happened to me and the fragments I remember. Polio fevers were generally mild, or in acute cases led to paralysis after a short intense fever.

There was only one fever. And the little boy and I shared it. One fever across time.

The only way I can make sense of my experience, unless I write it off as hallucination, is to return to Leila's comment on the phone

> *A **Vision Quest** is a rite of passage in some Native American cultures. The ceremony of the Vision Quest is one of the most universal and ancient means to find spiritual guidance and purpose. A Vision Quest can provide deep understanding of one's life purpose.*
> *A traditional Native American Vision Quest consists of a person spending one to four days and nights secluded in nature. This provides time for deep communion with the fundamental forces and spiritual energies of creation and self-identity. During this time of intense spiritual communication a person can receive profound insight into themselves and the world. This insight, typically in the form of a dream or Vision, relates directly to their purpose and destiny in life.*

in the hospital on the Night of the Blessing that my experience reminded her of a Vision Quest, a comment I couldn't assimilate at the time, but was starting to understand.

The Vision Quest was no head-trip.

It occurred to me that a person could be on a Vision Quest and not even know it, or experience it as such. I have some difficulty with the notion. The idea is taken or adapted from the native North American culture. Aren't we pulling it out of its cultural context, appropriating it even?

Maybe so. All crimes are possible. I'm just using whatever language, whatever notions are available to account for my experience. The language can never fit the experience one hundred percent. All cultural adaptions are improvised. There is leakage. Meaning suffers from its own form of entropy, and words grow shadows as if they were real things. My Vision Quest, was taking me back in time, or at least if the past cannot exist, into a realm where the little boy was still lying on a hospital bed in a

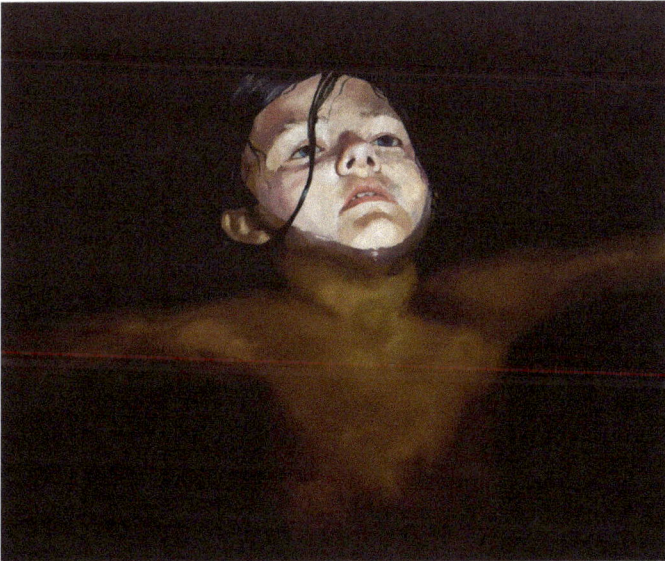

foetal position trying to be unborn yet too strong in the world.

Later, Leila was to tell me that I could have embraced the little boy and hence achieved a healing, but you can't make things happen in a fevre dream. They happen of their own accord or not at all.

An immediate issue when I left the hospital was if or when to take the antibiotics Dr Kali had prescribed. Common sense dictated that I should have taken them immediately, but that was not clear in the early days of the fevre dream. I had no abdominal pain. Aside from a general weakness that I ascribed to spending too long sitting on a hospital bed reading detective fiction and waiting for the tooth fairy of medicine to come by, I only had the temperature, which was almost sub-clinical most of the time, hovering at the upper edge of normal. I knew I was still anaemic, but just how anaemic I didn't realize at the time.

I felt very tired, very frail in the face of the material world. When I looked at my body in the mirror I hardly recognised myself. The trim, youthful looking man had been replaced by a gaunt, aged stickman. My veins stood out and my muscles could be clearly seen, muscles I'd never seen before. I had the scrawny arms of an old man.

You hear about people aging ten years in a few weeks, that's what it looked like. I had lost ten kilos, most of it in hospital. Whereas on my Saturday visit to Waiheke I had been able to walk with ease and enjoyment, now I could barely make it up the road to the corner. All my vital energy had been sucked right out of me.

I was sicker than I'd ever been.

I was beset by a constant awareness of the signs and symbols of the world, an over-riding sense of strangeness. My nightly visits to the hospital or the boy in his dream seemed out of proportion to the physical cause, a relatively slight rise in temperature, rarely above 38.5 degrees.

The decision with regard to the antibiotics was taken out of my hands. My 'team,' my guides, my inner promptings, whatever you want to call them, advised me to wait for 48 hours before taking the antibiotics. Since then I have often wondered about that instruction. In one respect my condition appeared to be stabilising by itself, and I deeply desired the recovery of my own powers for healing and regeneration.

On the very first night out of the hospital, at about 2am, my body went into a severe shaking fit. I was shaking like I was breaking, breaking apart. It began with the shivers and from the shivers to the trembles, and from the trembles to the shakes. Leila didn't know what to do except lie on top of me as if to quell the shaking by her very physical weight.

The next night the shakes returned only at a much reduced strength, and by the third night they had gone. We decided I'd suffered from, and might still be suffering from, a kind of post traumatic stress disorder. After all, my life had been blown apart just as surely as if a roadside bomb had exploded nearby.

There was a good chance that the associated weirdness of effect that I was experiencing was also an aspect of the shock reaction, and might in itself fade along with the elevated temperature – which I could control with paracetamol anyway if push came to shove, do what they do in hospital.

Therefore I was unprepared for the Day of Death, the second day of the 48 hours.

It began normally enough. My appetite was returning, a welcome development. My blood pressure was normal, bowels were coming into line. It was early in the day and my temperature was okay. The trouble started when I began to feel that it was very important not to see people, to not talk or have to talk, that was the instruction of the hour. I was to retreat. There was that same sense of urgency and busyness around me that I was experiencing at nights. The team was in crisis mode but there were no corresponding physical symptoms, at least apparently.

Not talking, not seeing anyone, was difficult as we had an occasional gardener doing some work around the house that day. It took me ages to get used to her, and to assimilate her into the gathering silence. The sense of withdrawing from people, from having to see people and talk and interact with them, was not a particularly pleasant one. The involuntary nature of it made it less than comfortable. Nor did it seem very spiritual in case you want to see it that way. Besides, there were implications. If I could be shut off from people I could just as easily be shut off from the rest of the world – as it so proved.

So, I found myself sitting in our living room not so much unable to move but with no reason to move. I wasn't hungry or thirsty, I had no body needs to attend to, so why get up and move around? I could read but had no desire to do so. I could listen to the radio, that most intimate of public media, but there was nothing on the airwaves but meaningless clatter. Clatter, natter, chatter. It was silence that I needed, at least as much silence as the world allows. Silence is an ante-chamber. Silence is endless, infinite. There is a silence so profound that no sound has ever reached it. Silence contains all sound. It is out of silence words appear and into which they vanish after being uttered. Silence haunts the words on the page, for they cannot live without sound, even imagined sound.

Somebody knocked on the door and a voice spoke. I recognised the voice as belonging to a Waiheke friend I'd known off and on for many years. He'd probably heard I'd been in hospital and had popped in to see how I was. There was no way I could talk, I was now in a place where there was no more talking. So I opened my mouth as if to talk and a voice came out – it was not my voice, not that I recognised.

'Please leave. I'm not seeing anyone.'

I could feel him hovering for a moment or two, indecisive, before moving off.

Shortly after that, I was instructed to go to bed while I still had the ability to walk. I checked my temperature. Barely over 37 degrees. Hardly panic stations. So I went and lay down. Almost immediately I felt physical energy drain from my body.

'We're shutting you down,' a voice said loud and clear in my head. I could just turn my head a little and see the pillow on the bed next to me, the sunlight coming through the window, the green of the trees beyond, a possibility of a sky, otherwise there was a shutting down alright – a shutting down of all movement. No movement could be willed. My muscles hung like limp sails with no wind to fill them. I was in my body but not of my body. It is difficult for me to write this because to write it I have to relive it, and it was a terrifying moment, at least in retrospect. At the time, however, I was not frightened, but was deeply amazed. This is very very weird, I remember thinking. I had no precedent in my experience for this.

'This is what it's like when it turns into paralysis,' the voice said. I understood that they were showing me something, something about the boy in the hospital bed with polio fever. That little boy nearly died. Or all the strength had been drained from his muscles and he was unable to move, like I was. This is what he fought off for all those weeks. This was the beginning of dying, the withdrawing from the body, the cutting off, the shutting down, the entropy, the dawning knowledge of that far off place where the stars go to die their soundless deaths.

I don't remember how it ended, or how I got back on my feet, but somehow the demonstration was over and I was walking around.

Leila saw me shortly afterwards and described me as autistic. I was here, but barely. I'd come back. The world was familiar, but I was unfamiliar to the world. I put my foot down carefully as if I might sink right through the earth. I could feel the sun but it didn't warm me.

I gathered sticks for a fire.

The south wind blew.

The south wind blew right through my body.

There was a woman on the path watching me. I smiled at her.

I could poke a stick through the world.

At that moment, Leila thought I was dying.

I was dying. I was just this side of death.

I made a fire.

I tried to get warm, but my body had no power to generate heat.

I ate but the food was of a different substance to my body.

That night, when I might have hoped for some sleep, a new problem appeared or rather came to the fore. The urgent call to pee in the night followed by a lethargic dribble with some discomfort. By morning I decided to take the antibiotics. I couldn't risk the possibility of a urinary infection, even a low-grade one. Temperature or no temperature I couldn't eliminate the possibility that I'd brought something unwholesome back with me from Auckland Hospital. I was little more than a walking ghost. Maybe the antibiotic would put a little colour in my face, a little marrow in the bone. Maybe there was a pill that would restore the world to substance.

There was. A magic little pill called Penicillin. Within a couple of days of starting the Penicillin I began to feel better and more connected to the world. The fevre dream lifted. I was back in the land of the living, most of me, the parts that mattered. I was like a recovered zombie.

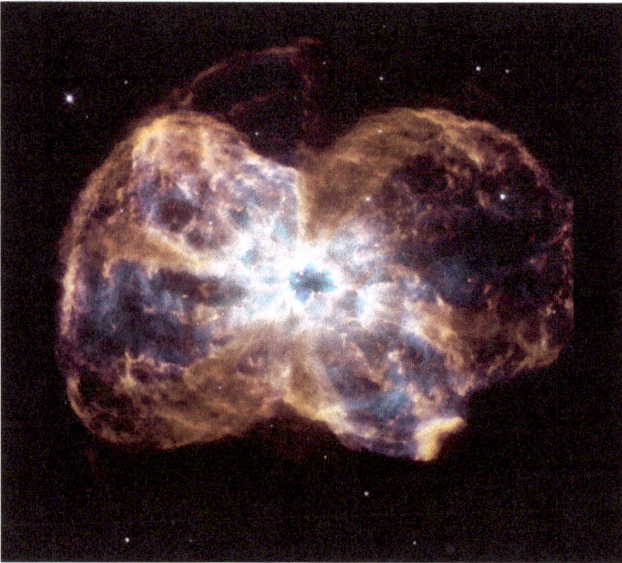

A Dying Star

'Now I can have a conversation with you,' Leila said with great relief.

'I'm back,' I said.

Things were looking up, at least a little. I began working steadily on this account, covering pages with my crabby handwriting. I was writing, and as long as I was writing I was alive. Soon I would be back to myself again, better than ever, bright-eyed and bushy-tailed. Yes, I had much to do! I had a story to tell. Words to write. Investigations to make.

It was almost like old times.

6

The Card Table

And so I hold myself back and swallow
My own dark birdcall –
Ah, where to turn?
Not angels, not men, and the cunning beasts
see at once that we are not reliably at home
in our deciphered world.

Rainer Maria Rilke

On the soft, green felt surface of the special card table with clever fold-out legs, three cards lie. One is face up, the Jack of Spades; the other two are face down, but I know what they are. The Joker and the Ace of Spades. The two cards have been turned face down but they have not been removed from the table. At any moment one or the other might flip over. Just like magic.

As I watch, another fourth card arrives face down on the soft green surface. I don't know this one. I want to turn it over and look. I don't want to turn it over and look. I'm frightened of what I might see. The hand reaching out to turn it over is not mine. It is the hand of an old man.

As the energy began to trickle into my body, I started to read more widely. Something happened to me and I wanted to assimilate it, reconcile it with my understanding of the world. I came across the writing of Miriam Greenspan, who, in *Healing Through the*

Dark Emotions, suggests that some illnesses might be a response to bad news we cannot handle any other way. Since the bad news cannot be assimilated emotionally, it may be discharged through the body.

Greenspan's symptoms are uncannily close to mine. She describes her research into what she calls emotional ecology, 'I was looking at how large emotional currents move through world events; how the environmental crisis and mass violence affect our emotional lives.'

I kept this up for a year, at which time I had a kind of breakdown of my own – more physical than mental. But clearly there was a mind/body relationship here. For months I'd been experiencing increasing stomach pain. I paid it no mind and continued my obsessive vigil of world events. It wasn't until I was literally on the floor in intractable pain that it occurred to me to have this thing looked into.

A series of tests told me that I had acute inflammation throughout my gastrointewstinal tract. I could no longer eat without pain. In fact I was in pain most of the time, but particularly just before, during and after a meal. I became averse to eating. What little food I did take in was poorly absorbed, so I grew weaker. My energy level declined alarmingly until I could barely walk... I'd forgotten the first and most essential skill of emotional alchemy: attending to emotional energy with awareness. As a result I lost my balance. Along with my cereal I imbibed the tears and blood, loneliness misery, trauma and horror that is daily life for millions of people on the planet. In the telling language of the body-metaphor, I "couldn't stomach" the pain of the world. I was not alchemising the dark emotions, I was swallowing them whole.

Miriam Greenspan, *Healing Through the Dark Emotions,*
2003

After accumulating bad news stories over a year, often taking them in with her morning breakfast, physical symptoms set in.

Our language reflects this mind-gut relationship in a variety of ways. We say sadness or some like emotion will 'kick us in the gut' and 'I've had a gutsful', and it's a 'pain in the guts' just thinking about it. It's enough to 'give you the shits.' Particularly when your gut 'clenches with fear.'

> *I paced the room waiting for his call, the feeling of anxiety churning in my stomach like something alive.*
>
> Michael Connelly, *The Poet*

The similarities to my own case, however, go deeper than the symptoms. In the year leading up to the illness, I had failed to follow through on an environmental project, partly because of my work load, but more because I found not just the information, the facts themselves, highly disturbing, 'gut wrenching' in their implications, and found the cognitive dissonance evident in our

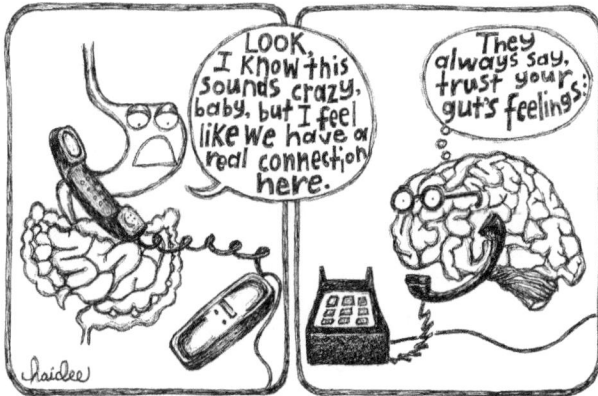

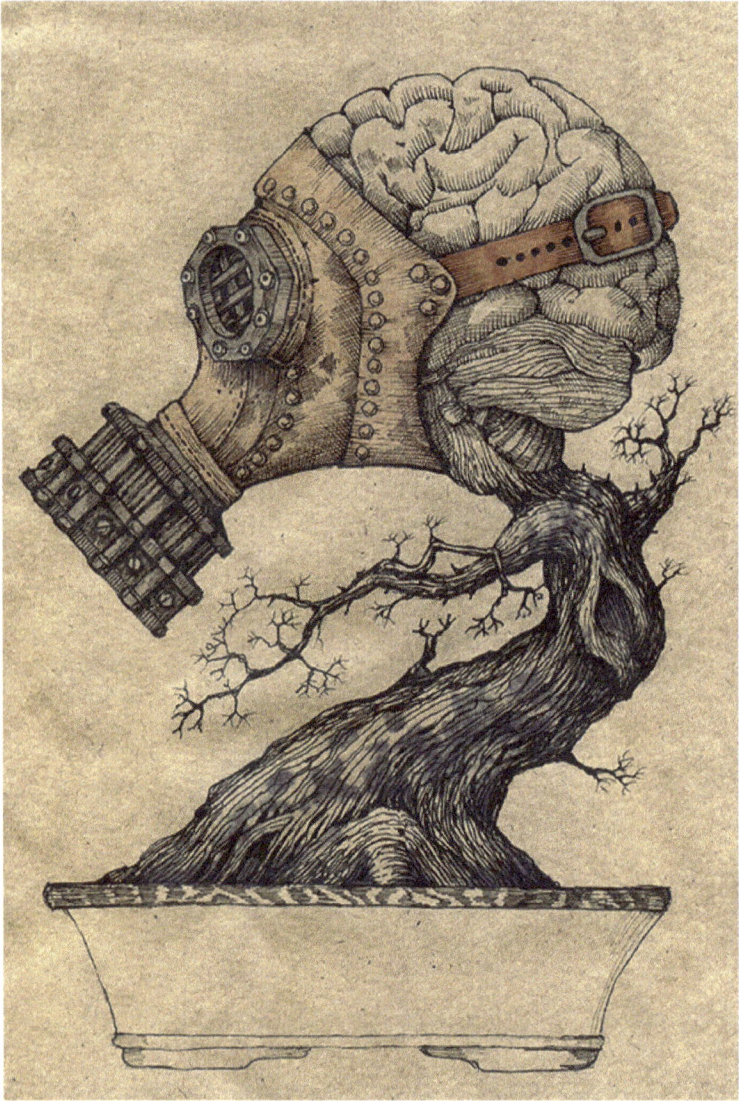

collective response to pollution and global warming frustrating in the extreme. It 'churned me up.' What do you do with a government that acknowledges the threat of global warming on one hand, while pushing the sale of coal, the dirtiest of the greenhouse gas emitters, on the other?

The destruction of the climatic conditions of the Holocene, which has nurtured humanity for the past ten thousand years is, quite literally, a sickening spectacle. It is like being forced to watch somebody you love commit suicide by self-poisoning. In the face of this ultimate challenge to our carbon consuming culture, we are reverting to fear and superstition. As a culture, we are closing down, regressing.

We can't handle the bad news.

These larger, cultural currents run through all of us. I certainly wouldn't be the first to be 'made sick' by the sight of environmental destruction. After all, the separation between a creature and its environment is, once again, an illusion, a convenience of language. Wound one and you wound the other. If the world bleeds I bleed. To attempt to live as if we were separate is in itself an illness. We are busy trying to 'cure' our psyche's attempts to heal the pain of that separation.

What is known as the 'mind-body and mind-gut connection' in Inflammatory Bowel Disease (the Ace of Spades) has a wider application to the mind-body relationship. A strict separation between mind and body is no more sustainable than the separation between electricity and magnetism, time and space. Just as the term spacetime has come into use, so has mind-body. We are no longer bodies living in space and subject to time, the classical view, but rather mind-bodies living in spacetime. A space-time-mind-body is what we are.

Just as the particle-wave duality can be dissolved by seeing

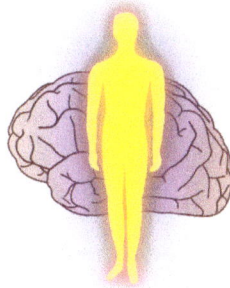

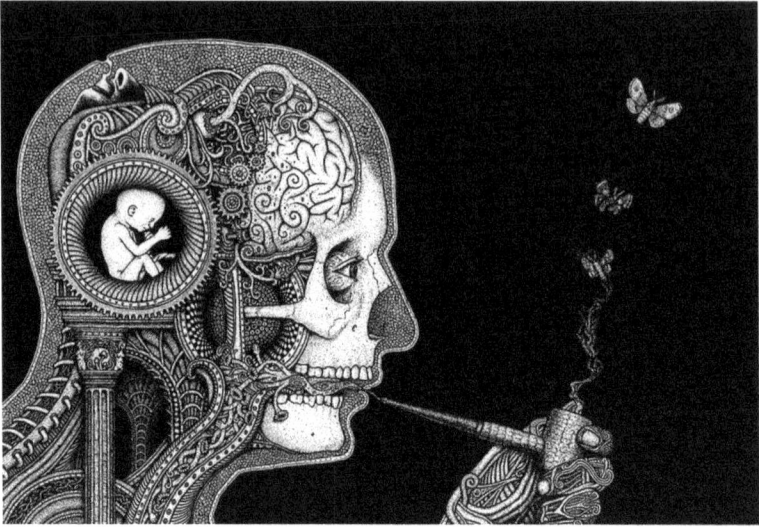

each as an expression of a deeper, underlying unity, so the mind-body duality can be dissolved in the same way – the underlying unity being called spirit. Sometimes I catch a glimpse of these multi-dimensional beings we call humans.

We only get glimpses, intimations. The rest is guesswork.

I did not, however, simply seize on this as the true and correct answer to everything. It sounded all very well, but what difference did it make in the end? And how was I to know? It was just another explanation in the mix.

A more fundamental problem, and one that soon became evident as the account grew, is how I could reconcile what had taken place with a rational view of the universe. I could see a tension emerging in the narrative between science, reason, and Leila's clairvoyant method. I wrote diatribes against 'reductionists' and 'rationalists' and crossed them out, making for ugly pages in the Moleskin Notebook.

The distinction between the natural and the supernatural isn't a natural one, but I lacked any theoretical framework for understanding that. The discovery of M Theory, therefore, I greeted with some relief.

> *In theoretical physics, M-theory is an extension of string theory in which eleven dimensions of spacetime are identified as seven higher-dimensions plus the four common dimensions (11D st = 7 hd + 4D).*

The eleven dimensions of M Theory are separate, discrete levels of existence, but they interact in ways we are only beginning to understand. The role that consciousness might play, within and across these eleven dimensions, is as yet uncharted by scientists. In a universe, or rather, multiverse, containing an infinite number of parallel worlds and a force we know as gravity leaking from another dimension into ours, what is not possible? Seven higher dimensions might just be enough to hide an angel, or Rilke's angelic order. Maybe even God is hiding away somewhere there in the maths, or rolled up tight in the superstrings.

> *This is not metaphysics. M Theory is the most complete mathematical description of the universe we have. In other words, without the eleven dimensions of M Theory we have no coherent way of making sense of what we observe in the behaviour of very large and very small things.*

I came to suspect that all this research, all this intellectual activity, was still a form of panic, albeit suppressed panic. I was seeking understanding and context, that was okay – but it seemed I was after more, that I was poking at the eleven dimensions in search of something else. Some hidden treasure. Reassurance – an after-life, perhaps? Perhaps, as with Sophia's Paleo diet, I was just grasping at straws with multipleworld theories and noble responses to world hurt.

Leila commented that I was being a bit hard on myself. Like my body, my bruised mind was trying to find its place in the world, to orient to the world as I was now starting to see it.

'You are returning to the world,' she said, 'but you are not the same person.'

It's not the same world, I thought.

'Return with the elixir,' I said, thinking of the final stages of narrative according to Vogler in which the hero, after battling his enemies and facing his demons, returns to his familiar world with his prize, his elixir of understanding. It might be treasure, it might be love. It was all about transformation and triumph. It didn't seem to have much to do with holding the line and trying to walk a little further each day.

In the meantime the medical profession had not gone away. They were as unhappy at the inconclusive outcome to their investigation as I was. Their answer was more testing. This time a magnetic resonance scan focusing on the liver. Whereas CT scans use X-rays, the MRI builds an image using radio waves generated by means of an electrical current and magnets. Everybody seemed to think that the MRI scan would be conclusive, definitive in some way. That it would finally clear up the mystery. More detailed images of the human body. Its results would trump those of the CT scan.

I was not so sure. More images on yet another screen.

Despite my assumed cynicism, I was still frightened at what the MRI might reveal. After all, my liver had had a long and chequered career, who knows what the images seen by the Science Fiction machine would show? I'd seen my liver in ultrasound looking like a mis-shapen pitted asteroid, subject to many a meteor shower. So I asked Leila if she would have a look a few days before the scan was due, maybe do any healing she could.

During this healing two things happened. Leila said she was shape-shifting into Snake Woman, a form in which she could enter my body. She related events as they went, how in snake form she was able to wrap herself around the liver and consume two black spots which she spat out. Then she sank deeper into the liver and was able to explore the internal structure of the organ, not just its surface. Her report was a sober one. There were darker areas of stagnant energy where the blood was not flowing easily. There was a sensation of heaviness and weight. Something unpleasant had taken root in the stagnancy, almost literally taken root, which had to be plucked out. Snake had to work hard to rip this unpleasantness

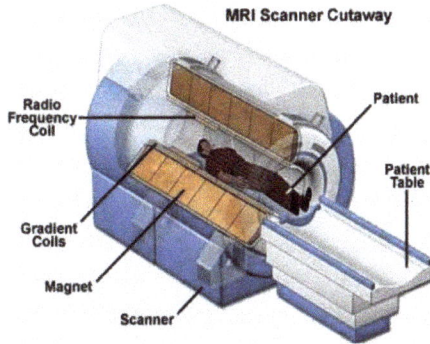

MRI Scanner Cutaway

Radio Frequency Coil

Patient

Patient Table

Gradient Coils

Magnet

Scanner

The mighty MRI scanner. A science fiction machine for the 21st Century, would not look out of place on the Starship Enterprise. I coped with the claustrophobia by tying a scarf around my head to cover my eyes.

Magnetic resonance imaging (MRI), is a medical imaging technique used in radiology to visualise internal structures of the body in detail. MRI makes use of the property of nuclear magnetic resonance to image nuclei of atoms inside the body. MRI can create more detailed images of the human body than are possible with X-Rays.

An MRI scanner is a device in which the patient lies within a large, powerful magnet where the magnetic field is used to align the magnetisation of some atomic nuclei in the body, and radiofrequency magnetic fields are applied to systematically alter the alignment of this magnetisation. This causes the nuclei to produce a rotating magnetic field detectable by the scanner – and this information is recorded to construct an image of the scanned area of the body.

out of the pathways of the liver, where it was like some kind of etheric didymo clogging everything up. I found myself working along beside her visualizing it as the work proceeded. Extracting that stagnancy was a protracted job.

Afterwards I could see how this work could exhaust her. I was exhausted too. Whatever it is that healers do might be a gift, but there is always a price to pay.

The problem with this kind of healing is that there is no way to verify it. A clear scan wouldn't prove that Leila as a snake being must have healed me. Maybe the illness was a clearing, part of the process of the liver repairing itself. Not an illness at all but a crisis brought on by a deeper healing process. I know some think this way, and good luck to them – I just didn't know.

As I had predicted, the MRI scan was inconclusive. It failed to find any lesions as such but did find 'patches of different density' which were a puzzle in themselves but apparently not malignant. Perhaps they were pre-cancerous spots. Or perhaps spots where cancers had healed. Or something else entirely. A new card on the table. Without the cancer hypothesis the medical profession was left without any explanation for the loss of red blood cells, the weight loss and the rest of it. Cancer was a nice fit.

Doctor Shiva was of the firm opinion that, cancer aside, I was not suffering from any Inflammatory Bowel Disease, like Crohns or colitis. He wanted to take the Ace of Spades off the table. The symptoms didn't fit. Janet was not convinced. What about those stubborn inflammation markers?

'I don't see how they can rule out IBD,' she said. She was not so much thinking of Crohns or colitis as diverticulitis, my Jack of Spades still face up on the table. If there were inflammation markers, the bowel was the best bet.

It was a big, unresolved mess.

In the meantime, my vital signs were slowly recovering. My red blood cell count was climbing. Inflammation indicators were down or steady. My appetite was good and I was putting on weight. There was every prospect of putting all this behind me.

'I think you did have cancer,' Leila said. 'But somehow you

threw it off. Your body threw it off.'

I wasn't so sure. I wasn't sure of anything. I didn't dare hope for anything. Not where the sly old Joker was concerned.

The 'team,' and the sense of being ordered around, had not gone away. The orders felt a lot more like guidance, although much of what I was being guided to do had no obvious meaning to me. For example, in investigating the liver I stumbled on the connection to traditional Chinese philosophy in which the liver is associated with anger – all the organs of the body are associated with emotions in traditional Chinese thought – and with the element wood, sometimes represented as a tree. Wood stands for springtime, re-generation, life, and I was immediately guided to a pine staff I'd had around for a year or two and which had never assumed any significance. Now it came to represent, even contain, the power of Qing Long, and I was to carry the staff around. Every time it hit the earth it connected me here, kept me here, on earth. The connection the staff made when it struck the earth would help heal me. Or not.

Then the axe fell. By a stroke of irony, or dreadful coincidence, I had a 'bleeding episode' while visiting the hospital for a catch-up consultation. I'd just finished having a blood test when I had the urge to go to the toilet. Out came the blood, thick and fast. I tried to keep my head and observe if it was bright red or dark. Bright

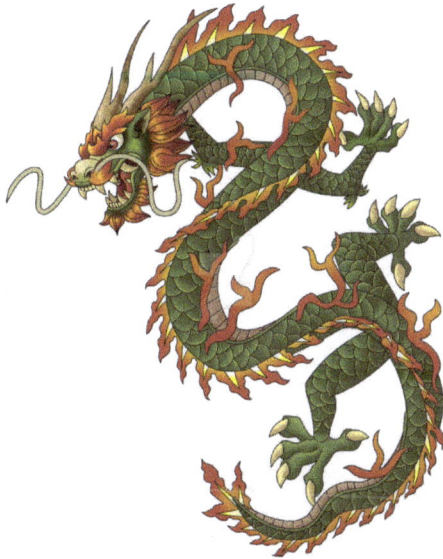

Qing Long – a powerful new ally? Or a fool's errand of the mind?

SYMPTOMS OF ANEMIA

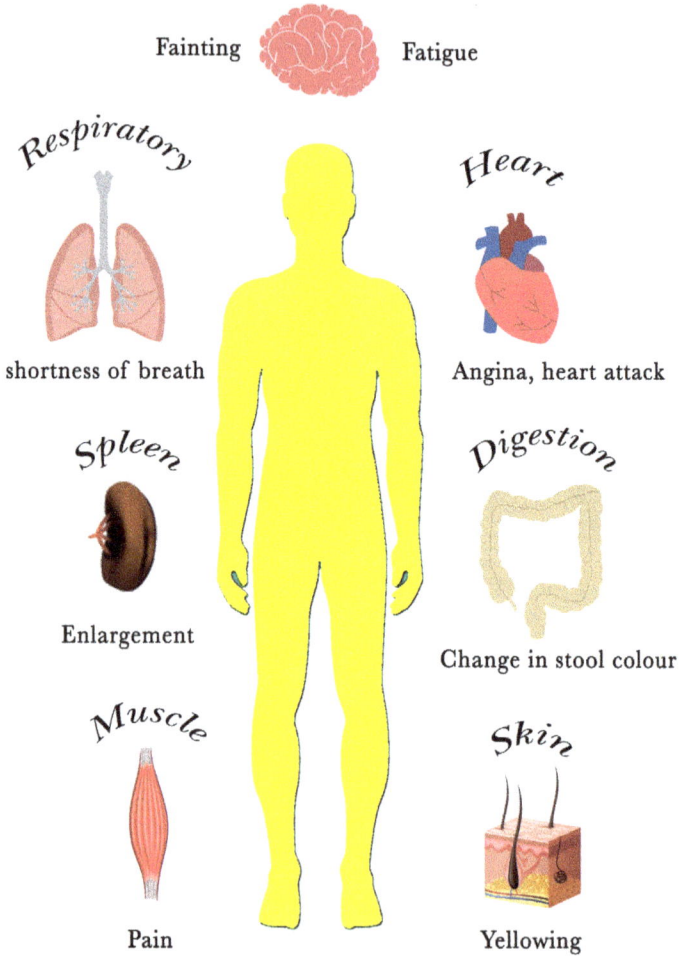

Fainting   Fatigue

Respiratory

shortness of breath

Heart

Angina, heart attack

Spleen

Enlargement

Digestion

Change in stool colour

Muscle

Pain

Skin

Yellowing

red, not so bad; dark, very bad. In fact it was both, mostly dark and slimy looking. Very bad.

I knew what this might portend, but had the presence of mind not to panic, to start shouting or yelling. Or getting a nurse. Show any nurse or doctor what I was looking at and I'd be back in Ward 61 before you could say colonoscopy. They'd be strapping me to a bed and slapping me on the drip.

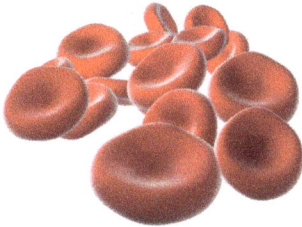

I'd grown too cunning for that.

I made it out of the hospital and into the park before vomiting. I vomited for half-an-hour, walking among trees – I probably looked like an old drunk. I felt like one.

'I must be allergic to hospitals,' I said to Leila later, having made it home. She tried to smile.

Unsurprisingly, my next blood test showed haemoglobin way

What does it matter now?
Only the next sentence matters.

I'm not lost, I'm here.

---

down. In red blood cell terms, I'd lost a litre of blood, Janet calculated.

'You're four points below the limit for me to order a blood transfusion,' Janet said.

'Is that what you recommend?'

'No. Because you're still walking around. You've had anaemia for years, I figure. Your body has got used to it. Functioning without sufficient oxygen. But it puts a tremendous strain on the body.'

She explained that I should not walk too vigorously as I would put stress on the heart, which would be faithfully trying to push sufficient oxygen into the body. Much of my recovery had involved walking a little further a little faster each day. Damned if I did, damned if I didn't.

A lot of the time I had to keep moving in order to keep breathing. I understood, however, that the cells of my body were asphyxiating. There were just not enough red blood cells to carry oxygen to every cell. Potentially, I faced another shut-down at any time.

'It's not over,' I said to Leila

'One day it will be over,' she said.

The surface of the card table is as smooth as velvet. The three cards are still there, the Joker, the Ace of Spades, and the Jack of Spades. Only the Jack is face up. The others seem to be waiting their time. I can see right through them. I know their faces.

Another card has joined the Three Illnesses, as I come to call them. I don't know what this card is. It is opaque. Another illness. Redemption. The morning star. The Void behind the Door.

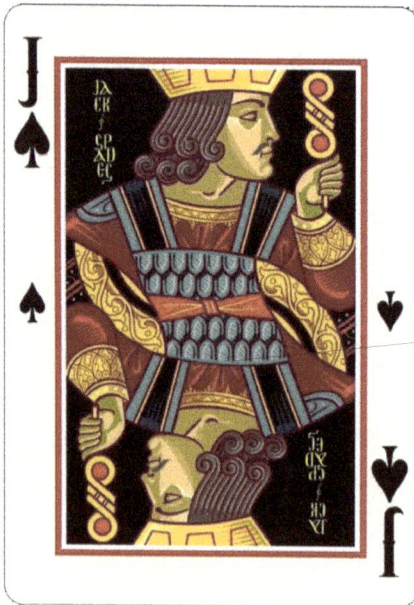

I see that I am coming to an end of the Moleskin Notebook, and feel the unease of shifting into the present tense. The past tense felt far more comfortable. The past tense is like a warm room on a cold night, the windows shut and curtains pulled. In contrast, the present tense is more scary, more open-ended. A sentence might begin and never finish.

As it comes to an end, I can see how the writing has supported me. On the very last blank side I scrawl a sentence. The next words write themselves. Only the next sentence...

Leila asks if I need a new notebook but after some hesitation I decline. It all fits into the hundred pages. There is something neat about that. The last blank page offers a closure that life doesn't afford until the very end. I can put a full stop at the end of the page, but I will wake up the next day just the same, alert and wondering. Waiting for the next blood test results. Watching for dawn. Watching for the next bleed.

Watching new light ruffle the surface of the card table.
I think I know what that mysterious last card is. Neither angel nor devil, sign or salvation. I can reach out and flip it over. An arm is reaching out to flip it over. The arm of a child.

This last card is blank. It has no face. Perhaps it is what I read it to be. Perhaps it outranks the Joker.   Perhaps it is nothing at all. A way station. Perhaps it hides secret words in invisible ink.

Or nothing more than the last line.

27th Oct 2013, Waiheke Island.

Illustrations and Quotes

Some chapter quotations are from Rainer Maria Rilke, The Duino Elegies, translated by David Young, the Field Translation Series, or A. S. King, and adapted by myself.

page 3:
The Angel of Compassion, Sculpture by Sharon Gainsburg

page 10:
How to Put on a Hospital Gown, sign found in the Auckland Hospital

page 11:
Healing Room, photo by Peter Rees

page 12:
What Leila Saw, watercolour painting by Leila Lees

page 15:
Alien, collage by D.G.

page 19:
CT Scanner, unknown artist

page 21:
What Leila Saw Next, watercolour painting by Leila Lees

page 22:
Týr and Fenrir by John Bauer, 1911

page 23:
Loneliness, unknown artist

page 25:
Eight of Diamonds, unknown artist

page 29:
still from Gordon Douglas movie *Them!*, 1954

page 40:
Michelangelo's *Image of the Face of God* from the Sistine Chapel, 1508-1512

page 43:
Playing Chess with Death, still from Ingmar Bergman's *The Seventh Seal*, 1957

page 47:
Michael Faraday lecturing at the Royal Institution of London, on his discoveries in magnetism and light, unknown illustrator, 1846

page 48:
Wave, by John Martin
Drawing of Albert Einstein by Subrata Dhar

page 49:
Photon Self Identity Problem by Nick Kim

page 50:
A Portrait of Space and Time (A Study of Existence) by Norman Duenas
Light and Dark, by Photoflake, Deviant Art

page 51:
The Orphic Egg by Jacob Bryant (1774)
The Multiverse, a page scan from *A Comprehensive Guide to Navigating Parallel Dimensions*, designed by Cameron Baxter
The Birth of Helen, Greek vase painting by Dijon, ca 375 - 350 B.C.

page 57:
Old Man in a Wheelchair, public domain, artist unknown

page 58:
Introduction to Gastroscopy by Dr. Hecker, in *Wiener Wochenchrift Magazine* (Nbr. 6/7 1896), illutrator unknown

page 59:
cartoon by Dave Blazek, originally published as part of *Loose Parts*

page 60:
nurse cartoons, originally published in Scrubs Magazine,

page 66: *S*
in Eater, originally published in Quanta Magazine

page 74:
Warning Exposed Void, recreated image seen at Auckland Hospital

page 77: c
artoon by Craig Swanson

page 78:
cover of *Operators and Things: The Inner Life of a Schizophrenic* by Barbara O'Brien, 1958

page 81:
A Little Boy Lost, illustrated by Dorothy P, Lathrop, 1920

page 83:
Black Pond II, oil on canvas, by Markus Akesson, 2013

page 88:
A Dying Star, image captured by the Hubble Space Telescope

page 93:
Brain- Gut, by Haidee Soule Merritt

Also by Mike Johnson

Novels
Zombie In A Spacesuit, 99% Press, Auckland.
Hold My Teeth While I Teach You To Dance. 99% Press, Auckland.
Travesty. Titus Books, Auckland.
Stench. Hazard Press, Christchurch.
Counterpart. Harper Collins, Sydney.
Lethal Dose. Hard Echo Press, Auckland.
Antibody Positive. Hard Echo Press, Auckland.
Lear: The Shakespeare Company Plays Lear at Babylon. Hard Echo
Press, Auckland (republished by 99% Press, Auckland).

Shorter Fiction
Confessions Of A Cockroach/Headstone, 99% Press, Auckland.
Back in the Day: Tales of NZ's Own Paradise Island, 99% Press,
Auckland.
Foreigners. Penguin Books, Auckland.

Poetry
Two Lines and a Garden, 99% Press, Auckland.
To Beatrice: Where We Crossed the Line. Pie Press, Auckland.
Vertical Harp: The Selected Poems of Li He. Titus Books, Auckland.
Treasure Hunt. Auckland University Press, Auckland.
Standing Wave. Hard Echo Press, Auckland.
From a Woman in Mt Eden Prison & Drawing Lessons. Hard Echo
Press, Auckland.
The Palanquin Ropes. Voice Press, Wellington.

Children's Fiction
Kenni And The Roof Slide, illustrated by Jennifer Rackham.
Beansprout Press. Auckland.
Taniwha. illustrated by Jennifer Rackham. Beansprout Press.
Auckland.

www.ingramcontent.com/pod-product-compliance
Lightning Source LLC
Chambersburg PA
CBHW052012030426
42334CB00029BA/3195